C B D HEMP OIL: THE MIRACLE HERBAL SUPPLEMENT

MEDICINAL HEALING AND HEALTH BENEFITS
WITHOUT GETTING HIGH

TERRY GORDON

© **Copyright 2019 by Terry Gordon / TGB Media Inc. - All rights reserved.**

This document is geared towards providing exact and reliable information regarding the subject covered. This publication is sold with the idea that the publisher is not required to render an accounting, officially permitted, or otherwise, of qualified services. If advice is necessary, legal or professional, a practiced individual in the profession should be ordered.

- From a Declaration of Principles which was accepted and approved equally by a Committee of the American Bar Association and a Committee of Publishers and Associations.

In no way is it legal to reproduce, duplicate, or transmit any part of this document in either electronic means or printed format. Recording of this publication is strictly prohibited and any storage of this document is not allowed unless with written permission from the publisher. All rights reserved.

The information provided herein is stated to be truthful and consistent, in that any liability, in terms of inattention or otherwise, by any usage or abuse of any policies, processes, or directions contained within is the solitary and utter responsibility of the recipient reader. Under no circumstances will any legal responsibility or blame be held against the publisher for any reparation, damages, or monetary loss due to the information herein, either directly or indirectly.

Respective authors own all copyrights not held by the publisher. The information herein is offered for informational purposes solely and is universal as so. The presentation of the information is without a contract or any type of guarantee assurance.

The trademarks that are used are without any consent, and the publication of the trademark is without permission or backing by the trademark owner. All trademarks and brands within this book are for clarifying purposes only and are the owned by the owners themselves, not affiliated with this document.

The information contained herein should not be construed as direct medical advice or recommendation. For medical advice, you should first consult your Physician.

Hello there my friend,

Thank you for purchasing my book. The content contained in this book will educate you on the health and healing properties of **CBD Hemp Oil**.

To add to your knowledge, I would like to offer you a free report that I'm sure you will find interesting. Simply click on the link below to access this **free report**:

"Healing with Herbs & Growing Your Own Herbs and Vegetables"

You will also be added to my advanced reading list group that makes you eligible to receive my upcoming new book releases prior to the launch date.

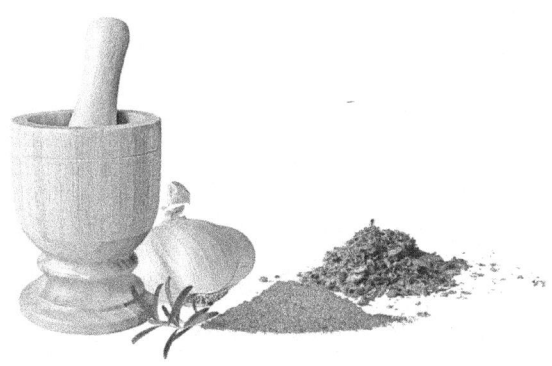

I would like to ask you for a favor. After you read this book, would you be kind enough to leave a review on Amazon? It would be greatly appreciated.

Click here to leave a review for this book on Amazon

Best regards,

Terry Gordon

TABLE OF CONTENTS

Preface	1
Chapter 1: An Introduction to CBD Oil	3
Chapter 2: Methods of Consumption and Dosage Information	11
Chapter 3: The Benefits of CBD Oil	24
Chapter 4: Buying CBD Oil	50
Chapter 5: Cooking with CBD Oil	60
Chapter 6: CBD Oil-Infused Recipes	64
CBD Butter	65
Golden Milk with CBD Oil	67
Chocolate Latte with CBD Oil	69
Chocolate Coconut Fat Bombs with CBD Oil	71
Peppermint Chocolate Cups with CBD Oil	73
Cookies, Cream and CBD Oil Cheesecake Bites	75
Chocolate Chip Cookies with CBD Oil	78
Guacamole Dip	80
Strawberry and CBD Oil Vinaigrette Salad Dressing	82
Strawberry, Orange, and CBD Oil Salad Dressing	84
Coconut Water Ice Cubes with CBD Oil	86
CBD Gummies	88
CBD Parfait with Hemp Milk	90
CBD Pesto Pasta With Shrimp	92
CBD Infused Parmesan Mashed Potatoes	95
CBD Infused Steak and Veggie Bowls	97
CBD Infused Mozzarella Stuffed Meatballs	100
CBD Infused Chicken Penne Alfredo	102
CBD Chamomile Tea Latte	104
CBD Golden Milk Popsicles	106
CBD Iced Coffee	108
CBD Margarita	110
Chicken Salad with CBD Lemon Dressing	112
CBD Chili Con Carne	114
CBD Brownies	116

CBD Fresh Mint Tea	118
Ch. 7: Pet Edibles and Treats	120
Peanut Butter and Honey Treat with CBD Oil	121
Grain-Free Peanut Butter and Applesauce CBD Oil Treats	123
Frozen Yogurt and Peanut Butter Treats	125
No Bake Coconut and CBD Treats	127
Sweet Potato and CBD Treats	129
Frozen Pumpkin and CBD Treats	131
Conclusion	133
References	135

PREFACE

Though hemp products have been around for hundreds of thousands of years, it was not until the last 30-40 years that scientists found a renewed interest in CBD oil and the way that it works. This research came following the discovery of the endocannabinoid system in the body, which works to encourage healing and overall wellness through the body by creating balance. The system was named after the cannabinoid receptors that make up the system, interacting with the cannabinoids produced naturally by the body, as well as those that you ingest.

CBD oil is not illegal in most areas, provided it has been sourced responsibly. This book will teach you all you need to know about sourcing it legally and where you can buy it, as well as what to look for in a high-quality product. You'll also learn about the many benefits of CBD oil. In recent decades, clinical studies and research have shown that CBD hemp oil works closely with your body to produce incredible results. This includes everything from managing the symptoms of heart disease and diabetes, helping treat pain, anxiety, and depression, and even fighting against severe autoimmune disorders, neurodegenerative disorders and cancer. As you read, you'll learn about what research is currently available that proves CBD hemp oil is effective in treating all these things and more.

Finally, this book will teach you what you need to know about the pharmacology of CBD oil. You will learn about the many ways that it can be ingested and its specific effects, as well as the dosage needed to create your desired benefits. CBD oil may be used to treat certain ailments and conditions. However, it is important to remember that CBD Oil is also beneficial for promoting overall wellness and therefore can be used as a daily health supplement to benefit anyone.

CHAPTER 1: AN INTRODUCTION TO CBD OIL

Advancement of medicine is a good thing. Surgeons and physicians can now treat conditions that they would not have been able to before. Through surgery, medicine, and various treatments, there is a way to relieve almost any condition. Unfortunately, all this advancement has also caused people to turn away from more natural medicine. Though Eastern medicine systems like Ayurveda and Traditional Chinese Medicine focus on all-over healing and the use of more natural healing routes, Western medicine relies heavily on solutions like surgery and medication.

This approach can be effective in certain cases. However, an alternative approach like that practiced by Eastern medicine systems has two advantages. When you choose a natural medicine, it typically produces several effects in the body. This encourages full-body healing and treats both the symptom and underlying conditions that may be causing the symptom. Natural remedies are typically milder in their effects on the body as well. This means that the condition, illness, or symptom can be treated without medication.

CBD oil works as a natural remedy would, causing full-body effects and treating underlying condition. Though there have been challenges surrounding its legality, this is not because of the CBD oil itself, but the stigma against the plant that CBD oil is derived from. Even so, more research has been conducted to discover the usefulness of CBD, which works with endocannabinoid system that already exists in your body. In this chapter, we'll take a look at what CBD oil is and its current legal status in the United States.

What Exactly is CBD Oil?

Cannabidiol (CBD) oil is derived from the hemp plant. Hemp is in the same family as the marijuana plant, however, its chemical structure is different. Marijuana is generally consumed for its medical effects and can result in a cerebral 'high.' By contrast, the benefits of CBD oil are purely medicinal. This is because the high association with marijuana comes from its THC (tetrahydrocannabinol). CBD oil does not contain any of the THC that causes a cerebral high. Instead, the CBDs work by activating the receptors of the endocannabinoid system. This improves your body's ability to heal itself, helps fight against free radicals that cause cancer and cell malformations, reduces pain, and so much more.

In most cases, cannabis strains are bred to be low in CBDs and high in THC. By contrast, hemp plants are high in CBDs and low in THC. Even though there are more than 130 cannabinoids that have been identified in cannabis plants, cannabidiol dominates the genetic makeup. Even though cannabidiol dominates in the oil, pure CBD oil also contains other CBDs that have been extracted from the plant, including omega-3 fatty acids, amino acids, chlorophyll, terpenes, vitamins and other phytocannabinoids, including CBC (cannabichromene), CBN (cannabinol), CBCV (cannabidivarin), and CBG (cannabigerol).

The Differences between Marijuana and CBD

When considering the legality, one of the major factors is the presence of THC in the CBD extract. The presence of THC depends on the genetic makeup of the plant. Some types of cannabidiol oil are sourced from hemp, while others are sourced from cannabis plants. The CBD oil sourced from cannabis plants contains many of the cannabinoids found in marijuana, with the highest concentration of CBD and THC. By contrast, CBD oil that has been sourced from hemp plants does not have the same high levels of THC. It is non-psychoactive, which makes it legal as long as there is no CBD. It also has the ability to counteract the effects of THC and has many medicinal benefits. Some people do choose marijuana-derived CBD oil because they enjoy the psychoactive effects. However, this is illegal in some states and countries because THC (marijuana) is illegal.

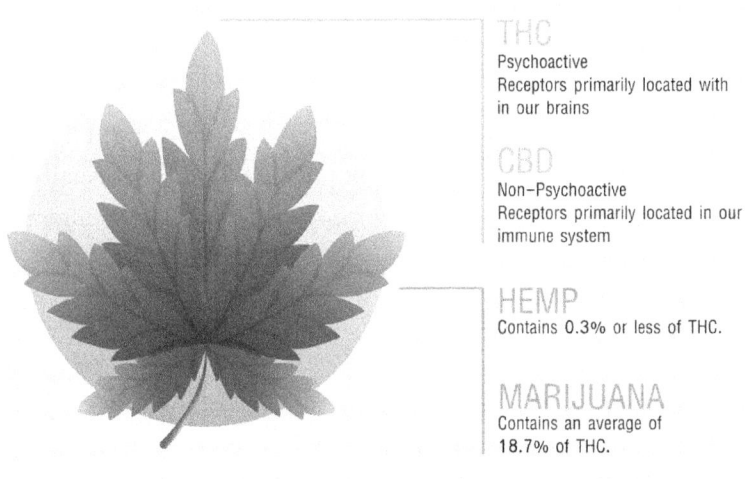

In recent years, many pharmaceutical companies have developed an interest in using CBD oil to treat pain, nausea, anxiety and other conditions, without the same side effects that are common with the use of many prescription medications. In some cases, CBD oil has been produced in a lab. While this is not as natural as CBD extracts, it does produce CBD oil effectively without the presence of THC. However, the downside is that many of the other beneficial cannabinoids found in the hemp plant are also not included in the extract.

How CBD Oil is produced

Before CBD oil is turned into an extract, salve, beauty product, or edible, the cannabidiol and other healthy ingredients must be extracted in a way that it can be added to various products. Typically, the flowers, stems and stalks of the hemp plant are used to create CBD oil. You should be cautious of companies that use the seed to create CBD oil extract, however, because the seeds of the hemp plant have a low concentration of cannabidiol. The extract will not be as potent as one made using the flowers, stems and stalks. The three most commonly used methods for creating CBD oil include alcohol extraction, oil extraction and carbon dioxide extraction.

Alcohol Extraction

Alcohol extraction requires alcohol with a high grain content like ethanol. Alcohol extraction is one of the less popular methods, especially since it destroys some of the other natural components found in the hemp plant. It is also one of the less efficient manners of extracting CBD oil.

The alcohol extraction method is most commonly used to create CBD oil tinctures. Tinctures are placed under the tongue to be absorbed or can be consumed in beverages. Essentially, the plant matter is soaked in alcohol for a certain period of time and then strained. As the plant material sits, the beneficial CBDs transfer from the plant to the alcohol.

Oil Extraction

Oil extraction has several benefits. It is a good choice for people who are processing oil at home, as well as companies who use oil in beauty products, supplements, or other applications. It is also easy to put in baked goods or other foods. This process requires plant matter to be covered in a carrier oil, which can be any type of oil. Some of the most commonly used are grapeseed oil, coconut oil, and olive oil.

As oil is gentler than alcohol, the resulting CBD oil has more nutritional components, which may have additional health benefits. Additionally, there are individual benefits from the different carrier oils that may be used. This comes from their high level of healthy fats and antioxidants, among other vitamins and minerals. The final benefit is that the resulting CBD oil is extremely potent. This is one of the most effective methods of extraction because the CBDs are extracted without resulting residue.

Carbon Dioxide (CO_2) Extraction

CO_2 extraction is most commonly used by companies that manufacture CBD oil, rather than people trying to make CO_2 extracts at home. This method uses a machine that forces carbon dioxide through materials from the hemp plant. This is done at a low temperature, instead relying on the high pressure to extract the cannabidiol and other oils, which minimizes waste.

The major benefit of CO_2 extraction is that it removes all the material except the beneficial ingredients including cannabidiol, phytochemicals, and other cannabinoids. CO_2 extraction also helps remove chlorophyll from the plant, which leaves behind a cleaner taste. Since the CO_2 method requires access to expensive machinery, it is not the most cost-effective way to create CBD oil. However, it is also very efficient, and the process does not leave residue behind.

The Legal Status of CBD Oil

The most confusion regarding the legality of CBD oil comes from its close relationship to the marijuana plant, which has been illegal at certain points through history. There have even been times in the United States where the growth and use of hemp were banned altogether, as politicians and researchers did not understand what each of the chemicals was responsible for.

At one time, it was said that any CBD oil was legal contingent upon the fact that it contained 0.3% or less of THC. There are even varieties that have 0.0% THC. These are legal to purchase and consume for medicinal benefits, even without any type of license. The confusion comes from the sourcing of CBD oil. In 2014, the Farm Bill was passed in the United States. This made it legal for hemp to be grown for academic research or under a state pilot program that allows hemp cultivation. As most of these plants are grown specifically with the intent of research and understanding more about how the hemp plant can be used, it is unlikely they have been sourced from one of these legal places. However, many companies have started sourcing their CBD oil from research facilities or hemp agriculturists outside of the country. Provided the content of THC is low, the shipments are legal to move across international boundaries.

Technically, CBD oil is legal in all 50 states within the United States, as well as various locations around the world. You should always purchase from a reputable company that has legal, ethical sources. Most companies will provide this information on their website or the bottle of CBD oil. Additionally, while there are a few select states allow for the growth of hemp plants as well as marijuana, where it is legal, most have not joined this stride. Unless hemp is legal to grow in your state, you should leave extraction methods to the professionals. Otherwise, you can still use CBD oil in salves, lotions and beauty products, as well as medicinally. The key is finding it sold as a dietary supplement, which makes it entirely legal.

A Brief History of Hemp and CBD

Though CBD oil is extracted from hemp, the plant also makes rope, fibers, clothing, sails, and more. It has been used many times through history in medicine and manufacturing. One of its earliest known uses was as hemp cord, identified in pottery that was discovered in modern-day Taiwan. This hemp cord pottery was estimated to be near 10,000 years old. It was a major part of agriculture and used around the world, with cannabis oil and seeds being used as food in 6000 BC China and hemp being used to create textiles around 4000 BC in Turkestan and China. In 2737 BC, CBD oil was used as medicine for the first time by the Chinese Emperor Shen Neng. From here, its medical use spread to India, with dried cannabis stems, seeds, and leaves (being called 'Bhang') were used as one of the five sacred plants of India, being used medicinally and in rituals. It was also used medicinally by Persians in 700-600 BC, as their religious text known as the Zendavesta refers to Bhang as a narcotic, meaning it relieved pain. There are many uses of hemp through history. Governments have traditionally encouraged this, with leaders like King Henry VIII fining farmers who did not grow hemp. The Puritans used sails made of hemp when they traveled from England to the United States. In the United States during World War I, farmers were given incentives to growing hemp, as it could be used for rope and other materials for the war. They could even use the revenue to pay off taxes owed to the government. By the late 1800s to early 1900s, CBD oil and hemp had grown in their applications. They were used in the automotive industry, to create building materials, and for materials like paper, plastics, clothing, rope and linens. Some companies even sold hemp products over-the-counter, both as medicine and in food products.

The decline came not long after, however, as companies started using synthetic fibers instead of hemp. These were easier to produce. Though this caused a sharp decline in the use of hemp, it was still grown by some farmers for its usefulness. This changed in 1937 when those farmers who still grew hemp had to pay to be licensed. The Marijuana Tax Act also required them to report any revenue and pay taxes on their hemp. Though there was a slight surge of popularity again in World War II, many farmers found themselves with canceled contracts by 1958 as the military no longer had a need for hemp. Soon after, hemp would become completely illegal.

Some credit Queen Elizabeth of England for the re-emergence of CBD oil usage, as she used CBD-rich strains in the 19th century treat severe menstrual pain. Regardless of the truth behind this, animal studies were conducted to understand how CBD worked in the body. Among the results of the studies conducted was evidence that cannabidiol has the potential to reduce the severity and frequency of seizures, treat pain, relieve anxiety, and more. The best strains were those that were low in the psychoactive ingredient THC and high in CBD.

Eventually, Britain-based GW Pharmaceuticals was given permission from the government to begin trials that would result in the first CBD extract oil. The goal was to create CBD oil from hemp that offered all the medicinal benefits offered from cannabidiol, without the psychoactive effects that result from THC consumption. Through the research of Geoffrey Guy and his team of researchers, GW Pharmaceuticals helped pioneer the use of CBD. Their research uncovered the ability of CBD to counteract the effects of THC, which could reduce the anxiety sometimes experienced by patients who used medical marijuana. Their research also uncovered many benefits of CBD oil, which offers its own benefits. After uncovering this research at a meeting with the International Cannabinoid Research Society, the team at GW Pharmaceuticals would work with HortaPharm to develop CBD-rich strains of cannabis that would provide the benefits of cannabidiol without the high. This was important because many of the seed companies working at the time were trying to grow strains of cannabis high in THC. As they worked with Robert Clarke and David Watson of HortaPharm, strains were developed that were high in the cannabidiol that produces the medicinal benefits.

Success would come around 2009 when cannabinoid-rich marijuana strains were identified by several dozen laboratories. As these strains were churned out, they were passed on to customers, including companies like GW Pharmaceuticals and other members of the International Cannabinoid Research Society. They continued their work and eventually produced legal medicine, with low-to-no THC content and a CBD: THC ratio with an average of 20:1. Over time, these would be used all through the CBD industry to create extracts, salves, balms, concentrates, edibles, and other CBD-rich products.

CHAPTER 2: METHODS OF CONSUMPTION AND DOSAGE INFORMATION

Though most people think of CBD oil as a supplement, it is available in a wide range of applications. One of the most common methods is smoking or vaporizing the CBD, as it provides the most immediate results. However, it can also be consumed in edibles, added to beverages, used as a tincture, and added to various topical products including creams, salves, lotions and beauty products. CBD oil is also found in capsule and tablet form, ideally used for people who want to take a pill with their daily vitamin and go on with their day. This chapter will break down the various ways you can consume CBD oil, as well as how to determine your ideal dosage.

Using Pure CBD Oil

The highest concentration of cannabidiol oil is going to be found in a pure oil form. It will not have any added ingredients or flavors and it is commonly processed using the CO_2 method. Without added flavors or ingredients, the taste can be off-putting to some people, especially if it is processed using alcohol instead of carbon dioxide.

As the taste can be off-putting, some people choose to add the CBD oil directly to a beverage or food, such as applesauce, yogurt or a smoothie.

However, when you ingest the CBD and it is processed through the digestive tract, the effect will not be as immediate or as potent as CBD oil that is administered sublingually (under the tongue).

In most cases, CBD hemp oil is sold with a dropper that lets you measure out an effective dosage. You control the potency by decreasing or increasing the amount that you take. As you consider CBD oil to purchase, keep in mind that oil is only the base product. In many cases, the CBD oil is sold a specific way, depending on the intended method of ingestion. You should always administer the oil according to the manufacturer's instructions, adjusting the dosage as needed. Some liquid applications are sold with the intent of being added to food or drink, while others are made especially for vaporizing. In some cases, CBD oil is sold in pre-measured applicators that let you easily administer the same dose every time without needing to measure. In these cases, you typically place the applicator under the tongue for a full minute before swallowing the liquid. This technique is used when an immediate and strong result is desired, such as in the case of relieving pain or stopping seizures. The area under the tongue is a direct route into the bloodstream, so it provides a powerful result.

Tinctures

Tinctures are commonly prepared using alcohol and are sold with a dropper or in pre-measured applicators. While tinctures can be eaten, the most effective way to administer them is by holding them under the tongue. Tinctures may also be used to create edible products out of cannabidiol as well. One of the major benefits of tinctures is that they allow you to control the dosage exactly, simply by adjusting the amount of liquid.

Unlike traditional CBD oil, tinctures come in flavored options that give it a better flavor. This is a good choice for people who do not like the grassy or chlorophyll-like taste that tinctures often have. They come in a wide range of flavors, including strawberry, cereal cinnamon, peppermint, vanilla, and more. Some tinctures are also sweetened, which makes them a good choice for adding to tea as well.

Tinctures are easy to add to beverages for people who do not want to consume their CBD oil in public. They also come in small bottles with an included dropper or pre-measured packets. These have the advantage of being discreet, so you can carry it around and use it when needed.

Capsules

CBD capsules contain CBD oil surrounded by gelatin, glycerin, or another capsule that breaks down once it passes into the digestive tract of the body. Since this method does not require you to measure a dose and it looks like any other dietary supplement, it is one of the most convenient and discreet methods. The capsules do not have an odor or flavor since they do not open until they have already been swallowed.

Another similar option is tablets, which usually contain a powdered form of CBD. Though these are sold as an alternative to capsules, powdered CBD does not have the same potency as CBD oil. It is generally processed more than oil, which reduces the number of beneficial ingredients. Additionally, the powdered CBD is not as easily absorbed by the body as oil, so you may need a bigger dosage and still experience fewer benefits.

The one downside of capsules is that they contain pre-measured amounts of CBD, so you cannot adjust the dosages in small increments. It is common for CBD capsules to be sold in a dosage containing 25 mg, though you may be able to find it in other increments. If you require long-term effects, such as people who struggle with inflammation, nausea, anxiety, or pain, this is a good choice because the effects last longer than when the oil is administered as a tincture. It is also a good choice for people who want to take CBD oil as a supplement since they can easily take their daily dose without having to measure their dosage.

Vaporizers

Vaporizers are a good choice for people who want to smoke their CBD oil.

This method has instant results since the lungs have a direct route to the bloodstream and they instantly absorb the CBDs as they are ingested. Some CBD oils come flavored, which can improve your experience.

For effectiveness when vaporizing oils, it's important that you choose a low-temperature vaporizer. You do not want to smoke the CBD oil but heat it just enough that it starts to vaporize. This will prevent the beneficial CBDs from being destroyed by the heat of the device. The most basic vaporizers look like an electronic cigarette, which makes them a little more discreet for use in public. Some devices require you to push a button as you draw in air to heat the oil, while others heat up as you take a breath.

Most vaporizers have at least two parts. One side contains the heating element and battery. These are made to work with a cartridge attached to a mouthpiece. In most cases, the CBD oil made for vaporizing comes in pre-filled cartridges. These are easy to replace, and you recharge the battery and heating element as needed. Some vaporizers do come with a refillable cartridge; however, you will still need to buy CBD oil designed especially for smoking.

Edibles

CBD edibles describe drinks, foods, and candies that are made using cannabidiol oil or tinctures. Unlike simply adding your own CBD oil to foods or drinks, edibles are made with the beneficial ingredients being incorporated into the edible. This allows it to be digested by the body more easily. Edibles are processed slowly by the body, creating effects similar to those you would get from taking CBD capsules. The beneficial CBDs are slow-released as your body digests, absorbs, and transports the cannabidiol to the different receptors of the body.

How quickly you will feel the effect of the CBD is not easy to pinpoint. Science dictates that, because treatments are consumed orally and must pass through our digestive systems, that it can take between six and eight hours for the edible to be broken down in the stomach and the small intestine and for all the available nutrients to be absorbed. The effects of the CBD in your chosen edible can last that long but you are unlikely to feel any effect for at least an hour after you consume it.

And, because CBD isn't psychoactive like THC is, it isn't always easy to produce a definitive result. You obviously don't get the high from eating a CBD edible that you would with THC but that isn't to say that it isn't doing its work. Some people have reported that, within an hour or so of eating an edible, they do start to feel calmer but, as with everything, that will be different with each person.

There are also some factors that can have an effect on how long CBD is effective for:

• When you last ate. How long it takes the edible to begin working and the length of time it will last will depend on whether your stomach is full or empty. If you ate a large meal not long before then the effects will take longer because your digestive system is still absorbing what you ate before. On the other hand, if you haven't eaten in a while, it will start working faster.

• Your metabolism. How and when nutrients from food are absorbed come down to your metabolism. If you have a fast metabolism, your body will process food much quicker and the effects of the CBD will start quicker. However, the effects may not last as long as if you have a slower metabolism.

• How strong the edible is; If the edible has a much higher CBD concentration, the effects may last longer. However, it is not recommended to take a higher dosage to make this happen. CBD tends to work better when administered over time, not all in one go.

What about dosage? As I mentioned earlier, you might not be sure what you should be taking so ask yourself what outcome you are after or what the symptoms are that you want help with. If you want a natural remedy for anxiety, for example, you won't need as high a dose as someone who suffers from insomnia. As with anything, start low and build up, especially if it is your first time.

Lastly, before you start buying and using CBD edibles on a regular basis you do need to be aware that none of the products available for sale have been through evaluation by the FDA and, as such, they are not regulated for medicinal use. While CBD definitely shows potential for alleviating some symptom, CBD edible may not be such a healthy alternative when you consider that they are full of sugar and other additives. So, before you go on a spending spree, so your homework and look for those that are made from natural ingredients and can prove that they have been lab tested and produced accurate results.

When you start to use them, make sure you pace yourself. Don't get trigger-happy and start eating too many. You need to wait at least half an hour and up to 90 minutes before the effects will begin and there is no point in eating more just to try and speed things up or make the results better. Start slow because, once the CBD is in your system, you cannot reduce it. If you need a faster way of ingesting the CBD, look into using vapes or tinctures; while these are effective straight away, do be aware that the effects will not last so long.

Many people have found that their health and wellbeing has improved dramatically by using CBD as a supplement but that is not a guarantee that consuming a CBD edible will make you feel any different. Every person is different in terms of chemistry and every person will have a different response to the next person. Do think about discussing this with your doctor before you start to use them, in particular if you are taking any prescription medications or have a pre-existing condition. While interaction is rare, it's better to be safe than sorry.

One of the downsides of edibles is that you cannot always tell how strong they are after eating them. Since they take time to be digested, you do not experience the effects right away. Additionally, you may be unsure of the size dosage you need the first few times. Something that can help is sourcing your CBD edibles from a company that is familiar with the potency of their edibles and can provide the milligram amount of CBD that you are getting per serving. Later I will give you a selection of recipes that you can make in your own home, along with helpful tips on cooking with CBD hemp oil.

Topical Applications

Topical applications of CBD include anything that can be applied externally. This can include CBD creams designed to treat eczema and psoriasis to pain balms and salves. Cannabidiol works better than other topical applications because of how deeply it penetrates the skin. This allows it to soothe pain and inflammation, as well as improve the overall health and smoothness of the skin. It also allows an area to be targeted specifically, providing more targeted relief. In some cases, topical applications are taken along with CBD oil capsules or tinctures. This provides targeted and general relief. Additionally, since topical applications need time to be absorbed by the skin (usually 1-2 hours), other methods provide relief while the topical application is being absorbed.

In addition to being used in medicine, it is not uncommon for CBD oil to be added to beauty products. The same nutritional components that promote health inside your body also nourish skin, hair, and nails. You can find CBD oil in shampoos and conditioners, lip balms, primers, lip balms, body mists, anti-aging products, soap, and other beauty products.

Something to note is that you may pay more for a topical product containing CBD oil than you would expect to. Though the base ingredients may be similar to other pain balms, salves, ointments, or beauty products, the addition of CBDs raises the cost considerably. A high concentration of CBD is required for it to penetrate the skin deeply and produce medicinal effects. Additionally, as CBD is considered a natural product, many companies choose to use sustainably-sourced ingredients, which can raise the total cost to make the product.

Dosage and Pharmacology

The specific dosage that you need for the effects of CBD oil to relieve pain, reduce anxiety, improve your overall mood, and create other desired effects depends on many factors. One factor is the severity of the condition. Someone who is taking CBD oil to promote overall wellness would need a much smaller dosage than someone who is taking CBD oil to reduce their seizures.

CBD Oil for General Wellness

In people who are trying to promote general wellness, CBD oil helps regulate sleep-wake cycles, regulate hormones, balance mood, improve immune response to illness, and improve pain levels. It also increases your ability to promote homeostasis in the body. This means in times of severe illness or traumatic injury, you have a better chance of returning to a healthy state. Even though your ECS is already functioning to promote balance in your body, giving it additional cannabinoids and increasing its number of receptors simply makes it work better.

When you are using CBD oil for general wellness, a tincture that contains around 2-3mg of CBD is ideal. You should start with a tincture because it allows you to make minor adjustments to the amount you are taking. An alternative to taking a tincture a few times a day is to start with a 25mg capsule of CBD oil. This will release slowly into the body and provide long-term results. It is also as easy to remember to take your capsule as it would be to take a multivitamin.

As you start your dosage, remember that it takes time before you feel the full effects, as you need to let the number of CB receptors through your body increase in number. You should wait at least a week after starting your dosage before increasing it at all. Additionally, you should always be careful that the dosage does not cause drowsiness each time that you increase it. Do not operate heavy machinery or drive unless you are sure it is safe to do so.

Other Dosage Recommendations for CBD Oil

People who wish to treat specific conditions with CBD oil should begin with a slightly larger dosage than people taking it for general wellness. For treating general ailments, a dosage of 5mg tincture is recommended twice per day. This can be useful for treating mood disorders like anxiety and depression, helping people who struggle with insomnia, and improving appetite control. For people taking a supplement, a 25 mg capsule should be taken twice daily instead.

People who are taking CBD oil for chronic pain should also start with a 5mg dose. This dosage should be significant enough that it increases your CB receptors. Then, increase as needed in increments of 5 mg, until you experience the pain relief you are hoping for. Though capsules can help with chronic pain and inflammation, tinctures are recommended because of their increased effectiveness.

Finally, people who are struggling with severe neurological conditions, seizures, multiple sclerosis, cancer, or other debilitating conditions should take a high dosage to help combat their illness. It is not uncommon for people with these conditions to start at a dosage around 80 mg per day, administered as a tincture. The amount may be increased depending on the effects.

To use topical applications, you should always thoroughly rub the balm or salve into the area where your pain is worst. You should expect to feel the effects with 1-2 hours. As manufacturers use different ingredients aside from CBD oil in their products, you should always rely on their instructions for how frequently the topical product can be applied.

Adjusting Your Dosage

When people do not experience the benefits that they are expecting from CBD oil, or they experience negative side effects, it is often the result of not using the right dosage. As every person's body is unique, it only makes sense that the ECS is unique as well. To find the right dosage, you must account for your body's unique ECS and take the time to adjust your dosage properly. There is no one-size-fits-all solution, as the way that CBD hemp oil interacts with the body is unique. Some people absorb the cannabinoids more easily than others, while others need a stronger dose to feel the same effects. Once you have regulated your dosage, you will experience relief from certain ailments and conditions, better mood, pain relief, and an improved sense of well-being.

Start with the base doses recommended above or follow the manufacturer's specific instructions. It is not possible to overdose on CBD oil; however, you may experience heightened drowsiness or anxiety if you consume too much. Give your body time to adjust to a new dosage before assuming that it is not working. If you feel groggy, reduce the dose slightly until you find a happy medium. You should always wait at least one week before increasing or decreasing your dosage, however, it may be better to wait 2-3 weeks the first time.

Are There Any Side Effects?

One of the reasons that CBD hemp oil has been considered a miracle drug by those who have learned more about its abilities is because of its incredible ability to treat a wide range of conditions. It also has minimal side effects, especially when compared to other pharmaceuticals and treatments commonly used in western medicine.

The side effects related to the use of CBD oil are minimal. The most common effects are slight drowsiness, dry mouth, and low blood pressure, which are much less severe than side effects of prescription medications. The amount of research conducted in the last few decades has tested the effects of CBD oil on several areas of the body. There are no adverse side effects in any of the following areas:

- Blood glucose levels
- Digestive problems
- Heart rate
- Electrolyte (potassium and sodium) levels
- pH levels
- Red blood cell volume

- The exchange of oxygen and carbon dioxide between the lungs and the blood

- Blood pressure

- Body temperature

In addition to how safe CBD oil is, many people wonder if CBD oil will cause a positive result on a drug test. Drug tests do not test for cannabinoids, as they naturally occur in people's bodies. However, they do test for THC, barbiturates, opiates, alcohol, and other drugs. As long as the CBD oil you have chosen does not have THC in it, there is no reason you should have a positive result on a drug test.

CBD Oil and Pets

As early researchers were still determining if cannabidiol and other CBDs were drugs or medicinal products, much of the research involved animals. As all animals with a vertebra have an endocannabinoid system, it can be assumed that CBD oil works similarly in pets as it does in humans. Since it is not possible to overdose on CBD oil, it is easy to administer it to your pet if they are suffering from a chronic joint condition, cancer, or even the decline that comes with age.

While research has shown that the psychoactive effects of THC can harm animals especially dogs, CBDs interact with their ECS system as it would in humans. It has been used effectively in treating conditions in dogs and cats. Typically, you should start with a small dose of CBD oil based on your pet's size. It is best to administer it in dropper form, sublingually, or by baking it into treats. There has not been enough research on the use of CBD oil in pets to determine an effective dosage, so it is best to consult with a CBD hemp oil specialist or a veterinarian that is open to holistic treatments. They can monitor your pet for changes, as well as provide guidance on how much CBD oil you should give your pet.

From what research has been done, the benefits of using CBD oil for pets are quite varied. The CBD from Phytocannabinoids, which are the naturally occurring cannabinoids from the cannabis plant, offer soothing and calming effects, helping to balance out health and wellbeing for your pet as well as helping to promote healthy joints and good digestion.

CBD oil has also been shown to help your pets with:

- Anxiety caused by separation

- General anxiety

- Appetite loss

- Nausea

- Pain management

- Seizures

- The side effects caused by cancer and some cancer treatments

- Bringing comfort and eliminating pain at the end of their life

All pet owners are right to be concerned about the possible side effects of any treatment given to their pets and that includes the use of CBD oil. However, to date, there have been no reports of any adverse effects of using CBD oil for dogs or cats.

CBD oils based on Phytocannabinoids are not toxic and they do not cause any psychoactive effects either. Although it is recommended to start with small amounts and build up, it really isn't possible to overdose a pet. The medical Phytocannabinoids do contain THC; in very small amounts this may be beneficial to some pets, but it isn't recommended. Too much THC can cause bad reactions, including overdose and static ataxia. Unlike the high that humans experience with THC, ataxia is neurological toxicity, causing dysfunction of the sensory system and resulting in a loss of coordination in the head, limbs, and/or trunk of the body. It is for this reason that it is recommended to use CBD oil developed especially for pets.

The Phyto cannabinoid-based oil can also be used safely with any other medication your pet may be on, over the counter or prescribed. However, you should consult your veterinarian before you introduce it to their diet.

When you do introduce it to their diet, because it is not a particularly palatable oil and your pet isn't going to like the taste, you should always use a carrier oil, such as coconut oil or bake them into treats and later I will provide you with six easy to make recipes for dog treats.

CHAPTER 3: THE BENEFITS OF CBD OIL

As researchers have continued to learn more about the way cannabidiol interacts with the body, they have learned that it works for much more than pain management and treatment of conditions like seizures and anxiety. In this chapter, you'll learn about exactly how CBD oil works in the body and the health benefits of CBD oil.

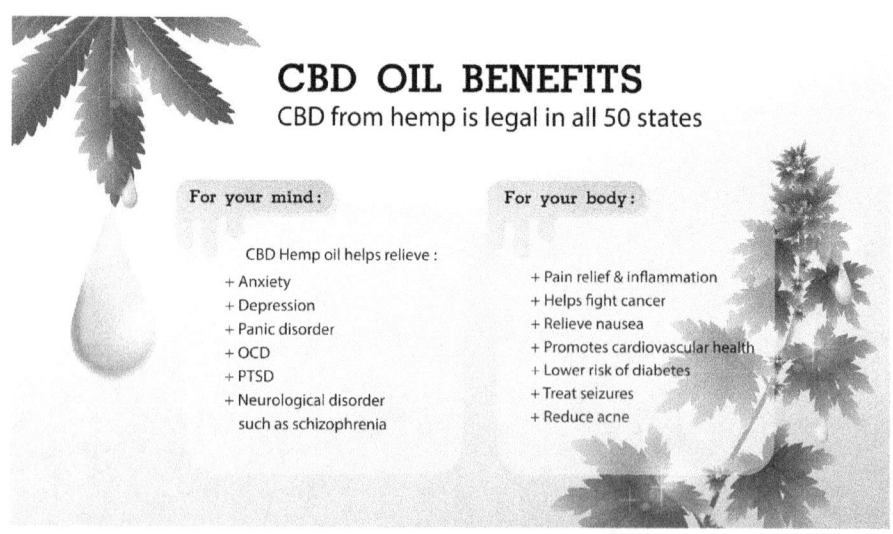

How Cannabidiol Interacts with the Body

The endogenous cannabinoid system (endocannabinoid system or ECS) was discovered in the 1990s, however, understanding this system has led to a much deeper understanding of how CBD works in the body. The ECS is a physiological system within the body that scientists believe may have developed as many as 600 million years ago. The system is made up of receptors that work with cannabinoids in the body.

Interestingly, most people do not experience their first interaction with cannabinoids when they use CBD oil for the first time. Rather, they consume cannabinoids that are produced naturally in their mother's breast milk when they are infants. The ECS is also not limited to humans—it has been found in pets like cats and dogs, and everything from nematodes and sea squirts to rats. If a species has vertebrae, research shows that it likely has an endocannabinoid system.

In each species that has been studied, the ECS is responsible for a similar task—maintaining physiological balance. This balance ensures that even when the environment outside of the body changes, the organism can continue living. By encouraging the physiological system to adapt to changes, the ECS may have even played a role in the evolution of different species over time.

What the Endocannabinoid System Does

You experience the ECS in action every day. Take a moment to think about how your body feels after you step out of a hot shower into a cool room. You feel cold, right? Usually, the longer you are in that cool room, the more your body adapts to the temperature. This is the ECS at work trying to stabilize the temperature of your body and make you feel more comfortable. The ECS is also responsible for critical activities in the body, including regulating sleep and appetite and promoting the healing of injured cells.

A Deeper Look at the ECS

The ECS exists in everyone, whether they have ingested CBDs in their lifetime or not. In this psychological system, there are two types of receptors that are called CB1 and CB2 receptors. CB1 receptors are found in trace amounts through the entire body. The greatest concentration of CB1 receptors are in the brain, however, they are also found in the muscle, fat, blood cells, immune system, kidneys, lungs, heart, and liver. The CB2 receptors of the body can also be found through different areas of the body. They are prominently found in the immune system, though they are also found in the muscle, liver, bones, and gut.

In people who do not ingest CBD oil, the CB receptors interact with natural CBDs that are produced by the body. Depending on where they are located, each receptor plays a specific role in creating homeostasis in the body. For example, when CB receptors in the immune system detect an illness, they trigger the body's immune response. This may cause a fever, which is intended to raise your internal temperature and kill the virus. Then, the CB receptors regulate the immune system, encouraging the communication between cells, tissues, and organs so they synchronize and balance as they were before the illness.

How the Body Produces CBD

Research on the endocannabinoid system has shown that anandamide, a neurotransmitter, is responsible for interacting with CB receptors through the body. The body produces arachidonic acid in the brain, which is the building block for anandamide. In addition to being produced by the body, anandamide is found in some foods, especially chocolate. This may be the reason that many people report eating chocolate makes them feel happier—it works with the pleasure and reward center of the brain.

Another role that CBDs play in the body is causing the egg to attach to the uterine wall during the reproduction process. It is unknown how else CBDs play a role in the reproduction process, aside from the benefits for babies are breastfed. In addition to being highly nutritious, breast milk contains cannabinoids. These improve a newborn's ability to fight off infection, encourage a healthy appetite, and improve digestion. These benefits are the reason that even when a mother is not planning on breastfeeding, doctors may encourage her to let the baby latch for the first few days, or even a few hours when it is possible. This is because the first few days, the mother produces colostrum instead of breast milk and the colostrum is rich with CBDs and other nutrients that encourage the baby's development and early nutrition.

Ingesting CBD: Why it's Important

You may be wondering why you should ingest CBD oil if your body is already producing CB receptors. Even though the body does naturally have these receptors, ingesting CBD oil programs your body to create more. CBD oil also has stronger cannabinoids than those that are produced by the body. This makes them more effective in triggering a strong response.

As new receptors are formed, the cannabinoids you ingest will start to interact with the new receptors. This causes them to become supercharged in a sense, giving them greater control over the body and their specific role in creating an environment of homeostasis. The cells gain the power to protect the body from harmful bacteria and viruses, fight against cancerous cells and malignancies, stop seizures, and much more.

Sometimes, people expect CBD oil to have an immediate result. Your body is not going to develop powerful, abundant receptors overnight. As you continue to ingest CBD oil, more receptors will form. You may experience some results the first time that you use CBD oil, however, the results usually increase over time as the body has time to create additional receptors.

Acne, Skin Conditions, and General Skin Care

The effects of CBD oil as an anti-inflammatory is one of the major reasons that it effectively treats skin conditions like acne, as well as more advanced problems like psoriasis, rosacea, and eczema. The redness, itchiness, and irritation of these conditions can be soothed by CBD oil. CBD oil also works to smooth the skin and increase moisture retention.

CBD oil can also be used in your beauty regimen to promote overall skin health and wellness. It helps plump skin and increases moisture retention, which can reduce the appearance of wrinkles and blemishes. As CBD oil can be easily added to hair products, moisturizers, and body washes, you can easily add it to your normal beauty regimen. There are also many CBD products available to promote skin health and wellness, including everything from healing salves and anti-aging products to pain balms.

Addictions

Even though marijuana has been called a 'gateway' drug by people who are against the use of the substance, research has shown this is far from the truth. Taking CBD oil has the ability to reduce the use of drugs and calm addiction in people who are struggling. Currently, research has conclusively shown that CBD oil can help people who are overcoming addiction to alcohol and cocaine, both reducing the urge to use and helping prevent relapse. This happens because cannabidiol interacts with the pleasure and reward center of the brain. It works by making the brain feel gratified, creating feelings of satisfaction even when alcohol or cocaine are not present.

ADHD/ADD

While people usually associate the symptoms of ADHD and ADD with being hyperactive, having an inability to focus, and being distracted, these symptoms are a result of low dopamine levels and high levels of cortisol. Cannabinoids work by trying to create balance in the brain, raising dopamine levels and reducing cortisol, which is a reaction to stress.

By calming the mind's reaction to stress, people struggling with ADD or ADHD can return their focus to the task at hand. Additionally, CBD oil can help reduce emotional outbursts that are common with these conditions. Among the studies carried out on ADHD and CBD use was a study carried out at the Nova Institute in Germany. Thirty patients with adult ADHD who were resistant to typical ADHD treatments were given cannabis. Some used it with their normal medication, while others only used the cannabis. Overall the patients experienced improvement of their symptoms, including an improved ability to speak without stuttering and focus on work and other tasks.

Age Related Macular Degeneration

Age related macular degeneration, or AMD, is a condition that affects people over the age of 50. It involves a loss of vision in the macula, the center of the visual field, which is caused by damage to the retina. It is considered to be an incurable disease and affects over 10 million people in the United States. While not curable, the degeneration can be managed or halted by several FDA treatments, ranging from prescription pills to injections directly into the eye. There are serious potential side effects when using these drugs, such as swollen eyes, sensitivity to light, infections of the eye, and even bleeding from the eyes.

CBD has been shown to have many of the same therapeutic effects as FDA approved treatments, but without any of the serious side effects. Because of CBD's anti-inflammatory and neuroprotective properties, it can improve eye health. It also has been shown to directly inhibit vascular endothelial growth factor or VEGF, a primary cause of AMD.

Alzheimer's disease and Other Neurodegenerative Disorders

People who develop Alzheimer's, Huntington's and other sharp mental decline have neurodegenerative disorders. These disorders are characterized by a progressive loss of neurological functioning, often causing lapses in memory and forgetfulness, emotional outbursts, psychotic or dissociative episodes, and other symptoms. The research shows that CBD oil can improve the symptoms in people with neurodegenerative disorders. While it will not stop the progression of the disease altogether, taking CBD oil has prolonged the lives of people suffering from Huntington's because it shows how quickly the disease progresses. In people with Alzheimer's, using CBD oil reduces the severity of frequency of forgetful episodes.

. . .

Anxiety

In the average person, anxiety plays a role as a critical stress response. It is part of our ingrained response that has existed since the beginning of man, as humans relied on it to be aware of their surroundings and quickly take in information to help them decide whether to fight-or-flight when they are in a dangerous situation. Even though it is a necessary part of the human stress response, some people are overly sensitive to their surroundings. This sensitivity results in anxiety, which can mean extreme feelings of nervousness for some people. For others, it can mean a rapid heartbeat, sweaty palms, or even hyperventilation.

Surprisingly, an estimated 18% of adults in the United States suffer from anxiety—that is about 40 million people. Though many pharmaceutical drugs have been developed to help with this epidemic, most of these come with side effects including decreased appetite, drowsiness, and more.

Cannabidiol creates a relaxed feeling. One of the reasons that people sometimes report feeling more anxious after smoking marijuana is because of the high levels of the psychoactive substance THC. Many strains of marijuana are high in THC, which creates the feeling of anxiety when there is not CBD present to counter-balance it. When marijuana is bred with a balanced ratio of THC-to-CBD, it allows people to get high without the feeling of anxiety. Therefore, by ingesting CBD oil alone, it can help people who already struggle with anxious feelings.

However, the key to an appropriate dosage for anxiety is taking the right amount of CBD oil. If too much oil is consumed, it can cause feelings of anxiety to return. It can even cause paranoia in some people. While many of the studies that have been done on anxiety have been conducted on mice, scientists have developed a deeper understanding of how CBDs may benefit people with anxiety. One way it works is by encouraging the brain to boost the level of serotonin stored in the synaptic space, which improves mood and reduces anxiety. It also works in the hippocampus by encouraging the birth of new neurons, which is critical because conditions like anxiety and depression decrease the number of cells in the hippocampus. This is the center of learning and memory in the brain.

There have also been studies conducted on humans. In Brazil, a double-blind study tested patients with generalized social anxiety. Patients were given CBD and most reported a significant decrease in the anxiety they felt. This was consistent with brain scans that showed improved cerebral blood flow patterns. Another study tested people with social anxiety disorder in a simulated test of public speaking. After ingesting CBD oil, most participants were less anxious—and their blood pressure and heart rate indicated their lower level of anxiety.

Arthritis

There are more than 100 different types of arthritis, with each of them sharing the common symptom of inflammation. There have been many studies conducted in lab rats that prove cannabidiol's anti-inflammatory properties are effective in treating arthritis and other joint disorders. The analgesic effects of CBD may also help reduce pain in these cases.

One study tested the effects of CBD on rheumatoid arthritis in mice, which is one of the most severe forms of arthritis. Marc Feldman of the Imperial College in London worked to find a dosage. With a few adjustments, the amount of inflammation in the mice decreased by an impressive 50%.

Bipolar Disorder

Right now, there are few studies showing the effects of CBD oil for bipolar disorder. However, what studies there have been have shown that CBD may generate the same or similar response as many, if not all, the medications that are currently being used to treat bipolar disorder. CBD has antioxidative and neuroprotective properties that may be able to help reduce the worst symptoms of the condition while increasing levels of BDNF (brain-derived neurotrophic factor).

There is plenty of testimony to be found from people who say that CBD oil has contributed to a high level of relief for their bipolar symptoms while reducing some of the side effects caused by the medication they are currently using. These testimonies are purely anecdotal but there is scientific evidence that backs it up:

- A research study funded by the federal government carried out a neurological assessment of 133 people who were all diagnosed with bipolar disorder. Each person was given 100 mg of CBD every day over a number of weeks and every one of them reported that their energy levels were consistent, and their moods were stable all day. When the study ended, neurological tests were carried out and all test participants showed significant levels of improvement in their verbal fluency, attention, functioning and in their logic-memory recall.

- Another research study was carried out on animals to study CBD antidepressive qualities. The research study showed that CBD had an influence on the levels of glutamate, cortical serotonin, and the 5-Ht1A receptors, helping to reduce depressive symptoms, as well as psychosis and also helped to normalize functions that affected psychiatric patients because of the way that CBD interacted with the serotonin receptors.

Research is also suggesting that CBD may act in much the same way as the antipsychotic drugs that tend to be prescribed for bipolar but without any of the long-term and serious side effects that can potentially occur. CBD does this through the provision of benefits related to mood stabilization and anticonvulsants as well as being valuable in use as an antidepressant that has little to no interaction with any prescribed treatments.

Bone Health

An estimated 8.9 million factions are caused every year as a result of weakened bones caused by osteoporosis. This condition is most common in the elderly, often leaving them fragile and susceptible to small falls that cause big problems. However, CBD oil may be able to help improve bone strength, both preventing bone diseases and helping brittle bones return to their original healthy state.

Many things happen to our bodies as they age. Bones start to break down faster than they can be rebuilt, absorbing too many vitamins and minerals that they cannot use. Your body also starts to produce high adrenal levels and more cortisol, which causes weaker bones. Since the production of these chemicals is common with aging, it explains why most elderly people experience lower bone density as they get older. Some other problems include the loss of collagen, which reduces bone mass and cartilage, as well as slower callus formation, which makes fractures heal at a slower rate.

CBD oil works in several ways to promote bone health. First, studies have shown that it regulates adrenal and cortisol levels, which is one of the ways that it helps to manage stress. Additionally, cannabidiol elevates the production of important chemicals in your body including collagen and boosts that absorption of vitamins and minerals. Finally, cannabidiol makes callus grow faster, which can help a fracture or break heal quicker after injury.

Cancer

Consider for a moment that over 600,000 people will die from cancer in 2018, according to projections by the National Cancer Institute. Many of these incidents are caused by exposure to unhealthy foods, ingestion of toxins, and lifestyle choices. Certain toxins cause cells to mutate and then attack other healthy cells in the body, resulting in the reproduction of cancerous cells and the spread of cancer.

Even though CBD oil shows promising results in slowing the spread of cancer, and possibly eliminating it in some people, no cure has been found that is 100% effective. The traditional approach involves having tumors (groups of cancerous cells) removed surgically or shrinking the tumor with radiation. These treatments come with many side effects, including nausea, hair loss, and a weakened immune system. The FDA has currently approved CBD oil for use in cancer patients to relieve the symptoms of their condition and the side effects of treatment, including pain and nausea. However, the most recent research shows promising results in the use of CBD oil to slow the progression of and even terminate cancer cells completely.

What is known about the way that cannabinoids fight cancer is that the goal of creating homeostasis encourages cancer cells to destroy themselves. When CBD oil is ingested, it increases the number of CB1 and CB2 receptors in the body. As these become stronger, they become capable of sending a signal to cancerous cells to destroy themselves.

The cells can be programmed to destroy themselves because of a process called autophagy. In a healthy body, autophagy happens constantly, as cells recycle parts of themselves to encourage the production of new cells and to keep the cells healthy. In the body of someone with cancer, the CB receptors program the autophagy process to destroy the entire cancerous cell, rather than recycling part of it. As the cancer cells are destroyed, damage to the surrounding cells is reversed and the body eventually achieves a state of balance. Of course, this is dependent on the progression of the cancer and how aggressive it is, compared to the level of receptors in the body. This has been effective in mice that were in a trial at the California Pacific Medical Center. The mice in the trial had either colon cancer or breast cancer. The results were astonishing, as a regular CBD regimen caused the cancer cells to disappear completely.

Chronic Pain, Joint Pain, and Inflammation

There are many causes of chronic pain, including conditions like arthritis, a failure of the body to heal after injury or genetics. Regardless of the cause, CBD oil has been proven to improve chronic pain. This is pain that lasts for a period longer than three months, whether it is constant, sporadic, or occurs after physical exertion.

CBD oil has anti-inflammatory properties that allow it to treat all types of inflammation, even when pharmaceutical treatments have failed. Some proven treatments include the use of CBD oil for multiple sclerosis and rheumatoid arthritis. It has also been used with success for treatment of pervasive muscle pain, migraines, and joint disorders.

CBD oil has also been proven to work for relieving pain. This often works with the same effectiveness, if not more, than traditional pharmaceuticals. Additionally, CBD oil provides pain relief without the risk of addiction and withdrawal that happens with the use of narcotics.

Even though CBD oil works better than some medicines for treating pain, the cannabinoids work in a similar way. Like typical OTC pain relievers, CBD oil works to relieve inflammation. It also interrupts the pain signal sent to the brain. For example, imagine that you fell and twisted your ankle. It is not the physical twisting of your ankle that hurts—but the signals that the neurotransmitters are sending to your brain. Pain pills stop the pain signals that are being sent to your brain, interrupting the pain you are experiencing. It also helps relieve pain by reducing inflammation. CBD oil also releases the neurotransmitters dopamine and serotonin, both of which play a role in your overall feeling of physical and mental wellness. This eases pain and discomfort.

Crohn's Disease

Crohn's disease is a variety of inflammatory bowel disease which most frequently affects the small intestine. Inflammation of the bowel is the primary symptom, which can lead to bloody diarrhea, fever, and abdominal pain. The treatments recommended these days can range from antibiotics to steroids and immune modifiers, all with potentially serious side effects.

A recent study attempted treating Crohn's disease with CBD oil. Patients that were treated with CBD oil experienced a significant improvement in symptoms. CBD oil has been shown to have anti-inflammatory properties, but there were other ways, not yet fully understood, that cannabidiol oil more directly worked to treat the Crohn's disease. Over 65 percent of the patients treated CBD oil met the criteria for total remission of symptoms, clearing up their IBD completely.

Depression

Depression is more than just a period of sadness. It often lasts longer than two weeks and can result in major changes, including a loss of interest in activities, changes in sleeping and eating patterns, difficulty making decisions, feelings of worthlessness, a constant feeling of tiredness, and problems concentrating. It is characterized by an imbalance of neurotransmitters in the brain, however, it is not necessarily these neurotransmitters at the root cause of the problem.

The balanced state that cannabidiol brings about in the body can help benefit depression. After CBD oil is ingested, it causes neurotransmitters and 'feel-good' hormones to increase in the brain. Specifically, it works with dopamine and serotonin receptors to boost pleasure and your overall sense of well-being. This creates an uplifting, positive mood that brings you into a balanced state. This helps prevent anxiety and stress that you may experience from life while relieving depression that you may be experiencing.

One of the studies that proved the effects of CBD oil on depression was conducted in 2011. While researchers were studying the serotonin system and its interaction with the endocannabinoid system, they uncovered evidence that proved cannabinoids regulated the stress response in the body. This led to the conclusion that in times of depression, CBDs may also help regulate your response to the stress of your daily life. With better reactions to stress, you may find your mood improves.

Diabetes

In people with diabetes, CBD oil helps lower insulin levels. One of the problems that people with diabetes have is that their body releases too much insulin when they consume carbohydrates, causing their blood sugar to skyrocket. If it gets too high, it can lead to coma or death. By reducing the amount of insulin that the body produces when you consume carbohydrates, blood sugar levels are lowered, and diabetes can be more easily managed. However, dosages are still being studied. As diabetes can be a life-threatening condition, you should never stop your prescribed treatments without speaking to your doctor. You will also need to closely monitor your insulin levels while using CBD oil.

Interestingly, CBD oil may also have implications in preventing Type 1 diabetes. Raphael Mechoulam bred mice, so they would develop type-1 diabetes around 14 weeks of age. In the first seven weeks of their lives, half the mice were given CBD oil and the other half were treated with a placebo. He would repeat the treatment seven weeks later. In the CBD group, only 30% of the mice developed diabetes, while the placebo group had a 90-100% development. Mechoulam was able to repeat this test with the mice again, this time introducing CBD at 14 weeks of age and testing at 24 weeks of age. Of those treated with CBD oil, only 30% developed diabetes.

Eating Disorders, Overeating, and Weight Management

When people think of using THC to get high, they often relate it to feelings of euphoria and developing the 'munchies,' which stimulates appetite. CBD oil also has an effect on eating, however, it can help create balance in the body. It encourages a healthy appetite, meaning it can encourage someone struggling with an eating disorder to eat and discourage someone who is overweight from eating too much. As CBD oil regulates the appetite, it triggers the release of hunger hormones. These help your brain know when your body is hungry and controls fullness and satiety levels as well. In addition to helping with the treatment of obesity and eating disorders, CBD oil may be used to increase appetite following surgery, after cancer treatment, or following a lengthy injury or illness.

In addition to being helpful in controlling overeating, research published in the journal Molecular and Cellular Biochemistry identified the effects of CBD on immature fat cells known as preadipocytes. The cannabidiol was proven to encourage the proteins and genes that break down and activate fat to work harder while boosting the number of mitochondria, which are directly responsible for how quickly the body burns calories. Cannabidiol also decreases the number of proteins in the body that generate fat cells.

Epilepsy and Seizures

Charlotte Figi is just one miraculous example of how CBD ingestion can improve seizures. One study was carried out by Stanford Medical Center, testing the effects of CBD oil on a small group of 19 children. Each child in the study suffered seizures that were both frequent and severe. In the testing group, none of the children had their seizures cease completely, however, 84% experienced a significant reduction both in the number of seizures and how severe they are. This research was incredibly important to the progression of the understanding of CBD, as a group of United Kingdom scientists began their work on a pure CBD extract following this study.

To date, several human studies have been done to test the effectiveness of CBDs in treating different types of epilepsy. One double-blind study tested a group of adult epileptics, finding that most patients experienced some type of improvement. About 50% of the group also stopped having seizures completely while they were taking CBD oil. Researchers have also come to understand how CBD interacts with different pharmaceuticals commonly prescribed for epilepsy and seizure disorders. It enhances the effects of some medicines while reducing the effects of others.

Cannabidiol reduces the frequency and severity of seizures because of its ability to calm and rewire the brain. It calms the receptors that are responsible for causing seizures in the brain directly. CBDs also have anticonvulsant properties, which stop spasms that happen in the body and mind. This works because seizures are caused by the brain working overtime, firing on all pistons and processing too many things at once. By calming down key areas of the brain, seizures are reduced. In some cases, it has even been said to heal epilepsy. It changes the proteins in the brain and rewires it, allowing it to form new connections that do not fire from the over-excited neurons. While this has not been tested in a laboratory setting, some people have reported being cured of their epilepsy completely after a CBD regimen.

Fibromyalgia

The pain of fibromyalgia is something that many people cannot see, as it affects the musculoskeletal system. Though it affects 5 million Americans, there has not been an effective treatment for this disease. However, cannabidiol oil has been proven to help people with fibromyalgia manage their pain levels and return to some functioning. It can also help improve sleep patterns, as people with fibromyalgia often suffer sleep disturbances because of their chronic pain.

Research conducted on the use of CBD oil on fibromyalgia has proven its effectiveness at more than relieving pain and encouraging rest. It can also manage symptoms including joint stiffness, anxiety, and depression. This allows fibromyalgia patients to return to some of their regular daily activities. A 2009 study also showed that over the course of 7 months, patients who used CBD oil reduced their reliance on opioids. This result has been repeated in several other studies as well.

Glaucoma

Glaucoma is a degenerative condition of the optic nerve, which often leads to partial or full blindness. Surprisingly, many people do not realize they have the condition until it is too late, even though the major symptom is worsening vision. It is most commonly caused by a variety of factors including ethnicity, age, family history, and underlying health conditions like poor eyesight and diabetes that can worsen your chance of developing glaucoma.

In most cases, people with glaucoma are recommended to take some type of eye drops, depending on the specific type of glaucoma they have. These eye drops relieve pressure on the optic nerve and help reduce the progression of the disease. Another possible treatment may be the use of CBD oil.

Surprisingly, the first study of marijuana use on glaucoma was conducted in 1971 by Hepler and Frank, who concluded that smoking marijuana reduced the pressure inside the eye by as much as 30% for 3-4 hours after smoking. Following this initial study, research has been done on CBD oil. It has also been proven to reduce intraocular pressure, thus slowing the advancement of glaucoma. This is due to the heavy presence of CB receptors found in the ocular nerves.

Heart Disease and Cardiovascular Health

Heart disease is the leading killer of men and women in the United States, often caused by a combination of poor lifestyle choices, environmental exposure, and genetics. CBD oil has started being recognized for its potential to treat heart disease and improve cardiovascular functioning, by lowering blood pressure, reducing arrhythmias, and relaxing the arteries.

Studies have shown that once the ECS is activated, it helps relax the arteries of the heart. It is known as a vasodilator, which reduces blood pressure, increases blood flow, and widens the arteries. As the arteries relax, they become less likely to develop clots as well. There is also a reduced risk of damage that can be caused by inflammation and swelling. Additionally, CBD oil often contains antioxidants that stop the oxidation of healthy cells in the heart. This was tested in a small crossover study, where nine healthy males were given CBD or a placebo. After just one dose, those who had taken the CBD had reduced stroke volume, reduced blood pressure, and better resting systolic pressure.

Researchers are still trying to understand how CBD hemp oil reduces arrhythmias. However, it may be caused by the CBDs interaction with the ECS. If the heart were beating irregularly, the ECS would try to create balance by sending the signal to slow or increase the heartbeat as needed. This has been tested in rats.

Research carried out at Hebrew University also showed an improvement in heart health following a heart attack. Mice who had heart attacks were given CBD oil. It reduced the amount of infarct, which is the amount of healthy heart muscle that dies after a heart attack, by 66%. With further research, this information could be used to reduce the mortality rate following a heart attack.

Finally, CBD hemp oil has been shown to prevent myocarditis, which is a serious condition that causes the heart to become inflamed. Once inflamed, the heart cells become damaged and start to die. This death can be caused by disease, virus, medication, or an attack by your own immune system. Untreated, myocarditis results in death. It is believed that CB receptors send out the signal to reduce the immune response to the heart, helping the heart muscle maintain its strength while inflamed. This prevents your body from causing further damage to your heart and reduces cell death.

High Blood Pressure

Formally known as hypertension, high blood pressure is a condition that affects millions of Americans. It most likely does not have one single cause, but it has been linked to high cholesterol diets, little physical activity, and even more nebulous aspects of lifestyle such as depression and economic status.

Even a single dose of CBD has been shown to positively affect blood pressure and patients' reaction to stress. The potential for it to reduce pain and stress is obviously helpful, but it may also have direct effects on the cardiovascular system that reduce blood pressure.

Immunity

There is a strong presence of CB receptors in the immune system, which helps create balance in your body and destroy viruses and illness. When you ingest CBD oil regularly, it increases the level of receptors and improves the functioning of your immune system. In some people, this boosted immunity allows them to treat exposure to allergens in their environment. Research has also shown the potential for improving the immune system in people who have autoimmune disorders or overactive immune systems. Autoimmune disorders are especially hard to treat and often require lifelong treatment of some kind, as the disorder causes the body to attack itself. By improving their immune system, these people find themselves less susceptible to illness and disease.

In people without allergies, autoimmune disorders, or weakened immune systems, CBD hemp oil can improve their body's overall immune response. This means that they may be less susceptible to illness. Even when they do get sick, people with a better immune response will not become as severely sick and their body can fight off the infection in less time.

Menopause

Going through the menopause is perhaps one of the most dramatic and significant times in a woman's life, not just because of the physical changes that her body will go through, but the mental and emotional changes too. The last time significant shifts in the reproductive system happened was puberty and these shifts can produce an unpleasant experience, including sudden mood swings, hot flashes, insomnia, and more. CBD oil has been shown to help in many ways.

We know that the endocannabinoid system is made up of a series of cell receptors that have the job of maintaining homeostasis and it is because of these receptors that cannabinoids such as CBD bind together and create the 'high' effects. However, the endocannabinoid system isn't just for cannabis; it is also highly interactive with the natural cannabinoids in the human body, the endocannabinoids.

The estrogen hormone is linked to this system through the regulation of FAAH, or fatty acid hydrolase enzyme, which can break down some cannabinoids. Levels of endocannabinoids and estrogen both peak when the other does and there is some early research to suggest that deficiencies in endocannabinoids may be the cause of early onset menopause.

There is also evidence to indicate that endocannabinoids are used by estrogen hormone to regulate both emotional response and moods, which does go some way towards explaining why mood swings are one of the most common symptoms of the menopause, at times when levels of estrogen drop considerably.

As such, it can be theorized that using CBD oil during menopause can help to shore up the vital functions in the endocannabinoid system that struggle when estrogen levels are too low. Although research is fairly scarce at the moment there are a number of ways that CBD oil can help to alleviate the symptoms, or at least significantly reduce them:

- Bone Density

Many women suffer from a loss of bone density when they go through the menopause and if it doesn't get treated, it can lead to something more serious, such as osteoporosis, not to mention other bone issues that can be debilitating, such as arthritis and rheumatoid arthritis, none of which can be cured. The hormone that helps regulate the replacement of the old cells in the bones with new ones is called estrogen and a significant decline in those levels will result in a gradual weakening of the bones. The cells that help break down the bones are called osteoclasts and bone loss is the result of the osteoclasts acting aggressively.

The osteoclasts contain untold numbers of GPR55 receptors and if these over-stimulate the cells then the bone loss will be excessive, which is what results in osteoporosis. There is research that indicates CBD oil can interact favorably with these receptors and slow down or stop them, reducing the risk of the bone density failing.

- Hot Flashes

This is another very common symptom of the menopause and they occur when heat builds up in the body intensively. It tends to start in the face and chest and is followed by alternate hot sweats and chills. Some women also say that, as it builds up, they feel more anxious.

Again, the anandamide, the natural endocannabinoid, helps to regulate the temperature in the body. CBD will help to raise anandamide levels in the human body by inhibiting the way that FAAH (fatty acid amide hydrolase). The effect is that women have a far better chance of being able to regulate their body temperature and the hot flashes will dissipate.

- Insomnia

When women suffer from insomnia during the menopause, it tends to be as a direct result of other symptoms, such as hot flashes, stiffness and pain in the joints and migraines; it isn't considered to be an actual symptom. However, if it isn't treated, a severe lack of sleep can lead to problems in other areas of life. It can also make the direct symptoms of menopause a good deal worse and lead to a worsening of mood swings or mood swings happening where they didn't before. There is quite a bit of documentation to support CBD oil as being effective as a natural way of helping to ease sleep problems. One of the properties of CBD is an anxiolytic effect, i.e. it promotes relaxation and inhibits anxiety, thus supporting deeper sleep and better rest.

- Pain Management

During the menopause, a number of changes occur in hormone levels and this can result in painful conditions arising, such as stiffness in the joints, aches in the muscles and migraines. CBD oil has already been proven to be most effective in relieving pain and is used the world over for managing pain in clinical settings.

There is research to show that CBD oil has a beneficial effect on pain and stiffness in joints and muscles and this is down to it inhibiting some of the cellular processes that result in pain and inflammation. The anti-inflammatory properties of CBD oil can help women going through the menopause go through their daily lives as normally as possible.

- Anxiety and Moods

When a woman suffers from mood swings during the menopause, it is a direct result of fluctuations in the levels of progesterone and estrogen and also tends to be joined by bouts of severe anxiety. It is no secret that menopausal women are far more anxious than those that are not going through it and much of this is down to the changes that they are going through, both emotional and physical. CBD oil has properties that can help to improve the mood and relieve anxiety.

There have been many studies on both human and animal subjects that show the anxiolytic properties and effects of CBD oil with the cannabinoid invoked for several different disorders, including depression and anxiety.

So far, research is showing that the part CBD oil plays in treating the symptoms of menopause is proving to be very useful as a natural treatment. There is still much research to be done but it is clear that CBD oil has a lot of promise and can also be used for treating symptoms of PMS and perimenopause as well as male menopause.

Mental Illness

In addition to common conditions like depression and anxiety, CBD oil has implications for the treatment of psychosis and schizophrenia. This comes from the anti-psychotic properties that cannabidiol has. Even though the idea of using CBD for treatment of psychotic episodes has been studied by scientists for decades, research has not yet been conclusive on what an effective dosage of CBD may be. Even so, the studies that have been done show that animals struggling with schizophrenia and psychosis show a positive correlation between the reduction of the severity and frequency of episodes. This theory hasn't been proven in human trials yet, however, there are anecdotes from schizophrenics who had their symptoms improve after using CBD.

Cannabidiol may help because of its antipsychotic properties. Like it relaxes excitable neurons in the case of seizures and causes new connections to form, CBD can help rewire the brain of people who have psychotic episodes. Something important to note, however, is that pure-CBD oils without THC content must be used by people with schizophrenia. Like THC can worsen the symptoms of anxiety, many people report that smoking marijuana causes or worsens their psychotic episodes.

Migraines

Migraines are not your average headache. People who suffer from migraines often suffer for hours to days at a time. Moving, being exposed to light, or hearing loud noises can all make a migraine worse. Some symptoms in addition to intense head pain and sensitivity to light or sound include nausea and difficulty seeing, driving, or concentration.

One study was published in Pharmacotherapy in 2016. The study took a group of 48 people who reported the use of CBD oil to treat migraines. Approximately 40% reported that the duration and frequency of their migraines decreased. Many others who did not experience benefits reported drowsiness following their dosage or difficulty determining how much CBD oil to take for the benefits.

One theory about the way that CBD oil works to prevent a migraine involves anandamide, a compound that helps regulate pain in the body. CBD oil stops the body from metabolizing the anandamide, which reduces the feeling of pain. Additionally, the reduction of inflammation can help certain migraines.

Nausea

Cannabidiol is non-psychotropic in nature, which defines medicines and herbs that have anti-nausea effects. It works by activating key auto-receptors in the body. As there are many conditions that cause nausea, including the treatment of cancer, pregnancy, and certain types of illness, there are many applications for nausea treatment using CBD oil. It is commonly prescribed along with traditional forms of treatment in cancer patients, to help negate the resulting severe nausea. However, as the research available on the use of CBD oil in mothers who are pregnant is slim, you should always consult with a professional before use. If your physician is not open to the use of CBD oil, you may find better guidance from a naturopath or homeopath specialist.

Parkinson's Disease

Parkinson's disease most commonly occurs in people over the age of 60. It is a neurodegenerative disorder that worsens with time, having symptoms that result in the loss of motor control, tremors, and trouble walking.

Many people with Parkinson's disease eventually end up in a wheelchair and it is not uncommon for depression to develop as a secondary symptom.

Parkinson's disease happens when the neurons in the brain responsible for developing dopamine start to break down. It stops sending dopamine as a neurotransmitter to the motor cortex, which results in the loss of function and movement. This happens as neurons are lost from the substantia nigra. In the early stages of Parkinson's disease, CBD oil is beneficial because it works with the plasticity of the brain to help re-wire the lost neurons in a way that ties motor function into the ECS. This is important because between 50 and 80 percent of neurons are lost before Parkinson's disease becomes apparent.

As the disease progresses, the dopamine neurons that are dying off start to develop a darker color. This causes brain cell death, as plaque builds up and the neuron is both physically and toxically obstructed. CBDs contain antioxidants that stop the oxidation of these structures and what is causing the plaque, which slows down how quickly Parkinson's disease progresses. CBD oil can also help with the psychological symptoms that result from the progression of the disease, by helping bring balance to the hormones in the brain and create a stable mood.

Sex Life Enhancement

CBD oil has been shown to have numerous benefits as far as enhancing sex life and one area where it has shown huge potential is in helping with erectile dysfunction. This is because CBD oil contains properties that help it to repair damage to tissues and improve the flow of blood to the genital organs. On top of that, because CBD oil can greatly boost levels of energy, it complements all the other effects vastly.

One recent piece of research showed that it is natural aging that causes erectile dysfunction because the process of aging results in a toxin known as dioxin being created. This toxin is directly responsible for erectile dysfunction, but CBD oil has been shown to flush dioxin out of the body, thus reversing the process.

The act of sexual intercourse may seem very simple, but it isn't. In technical terms it is quite complicated because, for a person to feel any desire, two systems in the human body need to be functioning properly. Those systems are the sexual excitation and the sexual inhibition systems, and both must work together to put a person in a desirable mood.

CBD oil assists both systems to work properly by creating a chemical reaction to reduce anxiety and stress. People who use CBD oil for this have reported that they can think a great deal clearer and have less nervous feelings, allowing them to express themselves in a better way. Not only that, by using CBD oil to create this, you get the same natural high without the need for psychoactive stimulation.

Some people, usually women, can experience some pain during sexual intercourse but CBD oil can reduce this or remove it altogether when it is used as a natural form of lubrication. Blood flow to the genital organs is improved and natural lubrication is stimulated, making things smoother and less painful all around. Plus, some studies show that when CBD oil is used as a lubricant, it can also increase levels of serotonin and decrease inflammation, both providing a person with more pleasurable feelings at the time of climax.

Sleep Disorders/Sleep Support

One of the common effects of THC is creating either a sleepy or stimulating effect, depending on whether the cannabis strain is indica-dominant or sativa-dominant. By contrast, many people turn to CBD oil because the amount needed to provide relief of pain, nausea, and other symptoms does not cause drowsiness. Even so, when ingested in large amounts, CBD hemp oil can have a sedative effect. Its ability to work as a sedative quiets the mind and calms the nervous system, helping to provide the relaxed state that your body needs to fall into a restorative sleep. This helps improve sleep patterns that have insomnia or difficulty sleeping as a result of other conditions, including post-traumatic stress disorder, restless leg syndrome, and interrupted sleep. Something to note is that when you take large amounts of CBD oil, it can cause you to become drowsy. You should not take a higher dose than you are used to and then use heavy machinery or drive, in case it causes drowsiness.

Stress

CBD oil is an adaptogen, meaning it helps the body maintain a state of balance during times of stress. It does this in two ways. First, it balances mental and emotional state by giving you the ability to relax and think more clearly. By overcoming anxiety and promoting a general feeling of well-being, it can reduce your response to stress in day-to-day life. CBD hemp oil is also an adaptogen that works to help you adjust to your physical environment. It is so powerful that researchers believe it may even play a role in the way that species adapt to their environment.

Over time, your improved reaction to stress will become part of your nature. Rather than panicking, your mind will get in the habit of rewiring your brain for a more appropriate reaction. You'll find yourself thinking clearer and making better decisions. This results from plasticity, which allows neurons to form new connections.

One study that tested this was published by researchers from Spain and Brazil and was published in Neuropsychopharmacology. A group of mice was put into stress for several days in a row. Two hours after the stress, the mice were given 30mg of CBD oil. The mice were also monitored for levels of neurogenesis. Over time, the mice continually increased their number of neurons, especially when battling the stress that they were put under. This shows how CBD hemp oil permanently changes your reaction to stress over time. Your brain forms new connections and new behaviors, which allows it to change in a positive way.

CHAPTER 4: BUYING CBD OIL

As CBD hemp oil has become legalized, it has become more widely available. At one time, people were limited to buying it from marijuana dispensaries or buying it online. While these are still an option, it has become more widely available. It may be sold at stores specializing in smoking products like vaporizers and tobacco, as well as health food stores. Some stores also sell it as a dietary supplement, recommending that it be used to promote overall wellness.

With so many options, it can be hard to decide where to start looking. Ideally, you should always purchase your CBD oil from a company with a good reputation and tested products. Since purity matters, you should look for a pure blend of CBD that does not have added ingredients. This chapter will tell you everything you need to know to buy CBD hemp oil, including general guidelines to follow, specific strains of hemp that are high in cannabidiol, and top brands that are currently available that provide great results.

General Advice for Buying CBD Oil

Most people who are buying CBD oil for the first time are not familiar with it. As not all brands of CBD oil are created equally, being familiar with what you are looking for can help you get the benefits you are expecting from the CBD oil. Here are some general guidelines that you should follow as you choose a brand. If you don't want to leave it up to chance, you'll find additional information on CBD hemp oil brands that have already satisfied many customers at the end of this chapter.

Look for Clarity of Labeling

Purchasing CBD oil should never be about guesswork. When a company does not have anything to hide, they will label their product clearly and ensure their customers have all the information they need to make a wise purchasing decision. Clarity says a lot about business ethics and the pride that a company takes in their product. If they can stand behind their product confidently, they will not use misleading or confusing labeling. As you look over the product, you should be able to find the following information:

- The concentration of cannabidiol and the overall purity of the product

- Information on how the oil was extracted from the hemp plant

- The name of the company that manufactured the oil

- The percentage of THC in the extract

- Basic dosage instructions (you may need to adjust these, depending on your condition)

In addition to looking for this information, the ideal company will have a label that reads 'GMP.' This label is a seal of approval meaning 'Good Manufacturing Practice.' GMP is a certification that is awarded to companies who have agreed to regular inspections of their extraction facilities. With the GMP label, you can be assured that the company you are buying from holds high standards for their CBD oil and creates consistent products.

Do Not Buy from Companies that Make Promises

A major red flag is a company that promises their CBD oil is a 'miracle' and it will cure 'everything.' Even though CBD oil has been proven to treat a wide range of conditions, the research has not been approved by the FDA. This means that companies cannot make guarantees of what it will cure. Additionally, as most CBD oil products are sold as dietary supplements, it is illegal for companies to make claims about what it can do medically.

When a company makes promises without having the research to support it, it may indicate they have not done enough research in other areas as well. The product they manufacture might not have a potent dose of CBD or it may not be manufactured in an effective way to provide benefits to consumers. Additionally, their dosage instructions may be inaccurate or unclear. The best thing you can do is choose a product that does not make these claims, but that has several other indicators that they have produced a high-quality product.

Where the Hemp Was Sourced

Not every hemp plant has been grown in the same conditions. Like with marijuana plants, hemp plants that have been grown in laboratories or in highly controlled settings are generally higher quality and more potent than those that have been stressed by an unpredictable growing environment. While this does not mean that people who grow at home or outdoors cannot produce quality strains, there is less chance of a low-quality product when the growing environment is controlled more closely. Laboratories and growing facilities often have better access to the equipment and technology necessary to create a better growing environment, though.

One of the biggest risks of low-quality grown hemp is that it may be exposed to pesticides and other toxins that may have been used to fight off insects, mold, or other common problems. However, hemp grown in a controlled environment can have a lower risk of being exposed to these things. For the highest-quality CBD oil, choose a brand that is certified organic. This means that the hemp has been grown naturally, without the introduction of toxins and man-made ingredients. Even though organic

CBD hemp oil will usually have a higher price tag, it is worth it since the goal of ingesting cannabinoids is to encourage health.

Select a Brand That Has Been Tested by a Third-Party

Third-party testing describes testing done by a facility unconnected to the company manufacturing the product. By choosing a facility outside of their control, manufacturers are ensuring the results are not skewed, biased, or tampered with in any way. The most common results of third-party testing will check the potency of a supplement and how pure it is. By submitting to this type of testing, a company is showing their faith in the quality of their own product. Other beneficial third-party tests include those that test for contaminants like heavy metals, mold, pesticides, and other substances. Even when you are buying a product in the store, their label should tell you if they have conducted third-party testing. You can usually find these results published on their website online.

As you consider the results of third-party testing, keep in mind that only the substances tested for can be identified. Not all testers will check for pesticides and other undesirable candidates. The only way to avoid these all together is to choose a certified organic brand of CBD hemp oil.

The Extraction Method Used

As discussed in Chapter 1, CBD oil can be processed using alcohol, oil, or CO_2 extraction. Sometimes, the process used depends on what the CBD oil is being used for. Alcohol extraction may be used in tinctures, while oil extraction is commonly used in edibles and beauty products. However, keep in mind that the purest and most effective method of extraction is carbon dioxide processing.

Regardless of the method used, it is important to choose an extract that has not been created by heating it to extreme temperatures. Heat destroys beneficial CBDs. This is the reason that people who choose to smoke their CBDs use special vaporizers—if the CBD oil is heated too much, it will destroy the beneficial ingredients. The vaporizers heat at a low temperature, which vaporizes the ingredients instead of burning them. When you are looking at bottles, you may notice that 'petroleum-free' processing is listed on the label. This is another term for carbon dioxide processing or CO_2 extraction. This preserves the most CBDs, however, it does also remove chlorophyll and some of the other beneficial ingredients. This results in a cleaner taste, though it may not have the same extra benefits that come from methods like oil extraction.

Find a Company with a Guarantee

While you do not want to buy CBD oil from a company that guarantees it will cure a wide range of ailments, you should buy from a company that offers a guarantee of their product. Some companies offer a money-back guarantee of some kind within a certain timeframe if you are not happy with the results of their product. This type of guarantee means that you are dealing with a company who values customer satisfaction over the potential of lost money. They believe their products will work and they stand behind that belief by offering a guarantee. However, keep in mind that the ease of the return process or money-back guarantee also reflects character. Some companies will require you to pay shipping to get a partial refund. In some cases, you may end up paying more to send it back than you would be refunded to begin with. Be sure to read the fine print and check a company's reputation before buying from them.

Choose a Company with a Solid Reputation

As dietary supplements like CBD oil are not regulated by the FDA, companies do not have to adhere to any specific guidelines. As long as their product has been tested for safety and it will not harm customers, it is legal to sell. This approval is only a guarantee of safety—it is not a guarantee that the product will work or that it has the potency it claims. When you are deciding to take something like a daily supplement, it should come from a company that has a solid reputation. Think about it like this. Would you buy a car from someone who has been known to cover up issues with their product, or who continues to sell vehicles when they know they are not up to the standard the buyer is expecting? Of course not. Likewise, you should not buy CBD oil from a company with poor practices or who has had problems with many of their previous customers.

Reviews of a product are one of the first places that you should look for information about business practices. However, keep in mind that not all companies will publish negative reviews if they have them. If reviews seem overly positive on a company's website, look at other websites and social media for reviews. You can also check with the Better Business Bureau. Here, companies receive grades based on the quality of their products and customer service. These claims are typically investigated, and companies are given a grade based on their quality.

Considerations when Buying Online

Some people do not have a local shop that sells CBD oil, while others want to use CBD discreetly. Even though it is legal and there is a difference between CBD and THC, those who are uninformed may still hold a stigma against it and people do not want to be seen using it because their neighbors, family, or friends will judge them. In this case, buying online is a good choice. However, to ensure the blend is legal, you must choose a brand of CBD hemp oil that contains less than 0.3% THC. Additionally, keep in mind that some companies offer discreet shipping if you do not want your neighbors finding out that you are using CBD oil.

Best Low-THC, High-CBD Strains of Cannabis

One of the major factors that affect the CBDs and beneficial ingredients found in a specific brand of oil is the strain of hemp that was used to create the product. Some products make use of the entire hemp plant, which offers additional benefits from cannabinoids other than cannabidiol, as well as beneficial vitamins and minerals. Others may use a laboratory to extract the cannabidiol. While this gives a higher concentration of CBD specifically, it also does not have the other beneficial ingredients.

The best choice is to choose a brand of CBD hemp oil that has been made from a quality strain of hemp. This information may be displayed on the website when buying online or on the battle. As research is still being conducted on the different cannabinoids and the effects that they have on the body, the best thing you can do is choose a high-CBD strain by looking at the information on the bottle. Keep in mind that the cannabidiol concentration is going to affect how potent each dosage is. However, even if a body reads that there is only 75% cannabidiol, it does not mean that it is not pure CBD. Most CBD oils contain cannabidiol in addition to other ingredients, which may or may not be listed. This includes other cannabinoids including CBC, CBG, and CBN, as well as compounds like chlorophyll, nitrogenous compounds, trace minerals, ketones, fatty acids, beta-carotene, vitamins, glycosides, pigments, flavonoids, terpenes, alkanes, amino acids, and water.

For a strain of hemp to be considered 'high' in CBD, it has to have at least 4% cannabidiol. However, most of the strains bred for medicinal use have a higher concentration than just 4%. With the research that has been conducted so far, some of the most beneficial strains for CBD extraction include:

- Charlotte's Web- Named after Charlotte Figi, this strain of hemp contains less than 0.5% THC—and an impressive 20% CBD. It was grown by the Stanley brothers in 2011. They originally developed this strain for cancer patients, however, their goals quickly changed when they saw the effects that it had on stopping Charlotte's seizures. The strain worked for Charlotte. However, there were mixed results on other children who tried the strain to reduce seizures. Currently, scientists in Colorado are trying to understand if there is a genetic difference that causes the strain to work for some children, but not for others.

- Avidekel- This strain contains an average of 15.8-16.3% CBD and has no presence of THC. This makes it ideal for people who want to try CBD oil, but who do not live in an area where marijuana (THC) is legal. This strain came to existence around 2012, bred by a government-licensed company named Tikum Olam. Since the strain has been tested on a wide range of conditions. It has been used heavily by Israeli patients and has also been tested at Hebrew University. Lead researcher Ruth Galilly reported that the studies showed a potential for treating inflammation of the liver, rheumatoid arthritis, diabetes, heart disease, and colitis.

• ACDC- This plant typically has around 20% CBD, with a ratio of 20:1 CBD and THC. It does not contain below the legal limit of THC, so it is not a good choice for people who live in states or countries where medicinal marijuana has not been legalized. Its high levels of CBD have allowed this strain to win the Cannabis Cup several times. It is ideal for treating anxiety and pain. Many people like to ingest this through vaporizing, as it as a unique sweet and skunky flavor. In addition to allowing relief of pain and anxiety, this strand is a sativa-indica blend that promotes both relaxation and focus.

• Harlequin- The Harlequin strain has 15% CBD, with a CBD: THC ratio of 5:2. Like ACDC, it is not legal to consume in all areas. This carefully bred strain is sativa-dominant and is a cross between Swiss Landrace, Thai, and Columbian gold. It is among one of the best strains for pain relief and has many anti-inflammatory properties. The research on this strain shows it effective at treating conditions that result in inflammation like arthritis and fibromyalgia. It also promotes an uplifted mood and can stop nausea symptoms.

Top CBD Brands Available

As the market for CBD oil and other hemp products has grown, there has been a surge in the brands offering 'high-quality' CBD supplements. If you do not want to do the research, be sure to consider these brands:

• PureKana Natural CBD Oil- This 99% pure oil offers full-spectrum benefits, which means the beneficial ingredients outside of cannabidiol have not been removed from the extract. It comes with a dropper to be used sublingually, which produces near-immediate results. The company uses hemp that has never come into contact with chemical fertilizers, pesticides, or solvents and is certified organic. They have also submitted to 3rd-party lab testing. PureKana has a solid reputation, being voted one of the best producers of CBD oil in 2017 and 2018 and being mentioned on major cannabis sites including High Times and HERB.

- Premium Jane CBD Oil- This is a natural, organic CBD hemp oil that is made in the United States. It does not contain preservatives or artificial flavors and has a full-spectrum of CBD benefits. Some of its natural flavors include vanilla and peppermint, which make it taste better when taken sublingually. This oil is also clear with its source, as all its oil has been sourced from the Kentucky Hemp Pilot Research Program.

- Green Roads CBD- This brand was created by pharmacists trying to create an alternative to OTC pharmaceuticals. It uses a highly-concentrated extraction process and full-spectrum benefits. Green Roads has submitted the 3rd-party testing. As an added benefit, their oil can be taken under the tongue or vaporized because it has a vegetable glycerin base.

- Charlotte's Web- This is oil made from the same strain created by the Stanley brothers. A major benefit of this CBD oil is that it has a specific line for dogs. It also comes in tasty natural flavors including mint chocolate. Each bottle has 500mg of CBD, as well as beneficial phytonutrients, amino acids, terpenes, and other cannabinoids. It is one of the most popular brands across the United States, likely because of its potency and its known ability to treat severe conditions like seizures.

- Hemp Bombs CBD- This brand is known for its potent dosage, which contains over 60mg of beneficial cannabidiol per dropper. It is derived from non-GMO hemp and contains full-spectrum benefits. It is especially beneficial for long-term use. They sell oils as well as vape liquids, many of them having an incredible flavor that sets them apart from other brands on the market. This brand is a good choice for chronic pain and generalized anxiety.

- Koi CBD- This brand excels in its wide variety of products. It contains pure CBD oil and is produced in an ISO-certified lab. It is known for being one of the cleanest oils available and is free of THC, solvents, hexane, GMOs, and pesticides. Among their many products include full vape kits, CBD vape liquids, sublingual oil, topical CBD applications, edibles, and treats for pets.

Keep in mind that this is not an all-inclusive list. As more brands become available and there are advancements in the way CBD oil is processed, prices are likely to decrease, and more companies may make strides toward entering the growing cannabis market. If you are going to stray away from these brands and try to find something locally or online, be sure to follow the tips provided earlier in this chapter to find a high-quality brand.

CHAPTER 5: COOKING WITH CBD OIL

Cooking with CBD oil is far easier than you possibly think it is and you can use it for anything, be it something sweet or savory. CBD oil is now one of the most popular oils because of all the properties and benefits it offers therapeutically, from managing stress and pain to clearing up your skin. You can buy CBD in several forms – pill, oil, or capsule – you can even buy CBD edibles but I'm going to be showing you how to make your own.

When you use the CBD oil in your cooking you get to determine how much (or little) you use, and you get to choose how you add it too. On its own, the oil doesn't taste that great but when you cook with it you don't even taste it. Before we look at some of the best recipes, here are a few tips to help you get started.

Sweet and Savory

Most of the recipes that use CDB oil and, indeed most of the edibles you can buy, are focused on sweet foods and baked goods and there is a reason for that. Sweet foods cover up the bitter taste of the oil much better than any other food, but you can also use it to great effect in savory foods too.

Before you can use the CBD in foods you must first infuse it with an oil or fat-based ingredient – this isn't quite so important if you are already using the oil in the first place. Some recipes also use alcohol instead of the oil or fat but do avoid using beer or wine – these are water-based and don't act as good carriers.

Temperature is Important

As far as temperature goes, CBD oil is quite fickle. While you can significantly increase the effectiveness of the oil by warming it, if the temperature is too high, you run the risk of some of the active ingredients being killed off. As a note to remember, CBD starts evaporating when the temperature goes above 320° F to 356° F.

Never, ever place the CBD oil over direct heat because the oil will lose its terpenes – these are the compounds that interact with the CBD to increase how effective it is. Plus, when you heat the CDB at too high a temperature, it gets more bitter in taste.

Start Small

It is all too easy to add a huge dollop of oil to your cooking when you first start. Not only can this lead to a waste of the precious oil, but it can also make the flavor very bad and you run the run the risk of overdosing on the effects of the compound. More isn't always a good thing, especially when you are a beginner.

Start small, in more ways than one. As well as starting off with a smaller serving of the CBD oil, make smear batches of each dish; if you like it, you can make more, if you don't, you haven't wasted much. You will also find it easier to get used to using the oil and the different serving sizes so that, in the future, you can make the alterations you need to get the most out of the dishes you prepare.

Storage is Important

Make sure that your CBD oil is stored correctly in between uses. It should be stored in a dark and cool place, preferably in a dark glass bottle.

Cannabinoids are extremely sensitive to light and heat and if not stored correctly, over time the quality of the oil and its potency will degrade. When that happens, the CBD oil is nowhere near as effective as it was and is likely to taste more bitter, leading to an unpleasant taste in whatever recipe you use it in.

Refined Oils are better

Choosing CBD oil that is more refined, is decarboxylated and/or filtered will serve you better for cooking with it. The oils that are not quite so refined will leave a bad taste in your mouth afterward, especially where your recipes are heavy on the herbs,

If you do only have a lower quality of oil available, you can still use it for cooking but only in dishes that already have a strong flavor to them, such as spicy foods or those made with chocolate. Plus, unfiltered oil contains more of the useful amino acids and vitamins than the filtered oils. Keep both – filtered and unfiltered – to get the best of both worlds.

Stir, Stir and Stir Some More

When you use CBD oil in your cooking there is one critical thing you need to remember – stir! Stir as much as you can because it is the only way to ensure that the oil is evenly distributed throughout your recipe.

It doesn't matter whether you are making a salad dressing, a batch of guacamole or a batch of cookie dough, stir more than you ever thought you needed to stir. That way, every part of the dish is equally as potent as the next one.

Cook Rather Than Drizzle

To get the best flavor, the recommendation is to cook with the oil but, should you be in a rush, there is nothing wrong with drizzling the oil over your meal – you won't get such a good taste, but the effects are still there.

Remembering not to overheat the oil, here are a few ideas on how you can use the oil:

- Add CBD butter to your toast, vegetables, potatoes or popcorn
- Add CBD butter to a cookie or dessert recipe
- Sauté your vegetables in the oil the same way you would any other oil
- Add CBD oil to salad dressings and sauces
- Add it to a pasta sauce – it tastes much better with creamy sauces
- Oven bake or roast vegetables and vegetable chips in the oil
- Use CBD oil in spicy dishes to ask the oil flavor
- Add it to a smoothie in the morning
- Add a bit to your nightcap in the evening – alcoholic or otherwise.

The possibilities really are endless; the most important things to remember when you use the oil for cooking are not to overheat it, start with small quantities and, most importantly, let your creative side out of the cage and have some fun.

CHAPTER 6: CBD OIL-INFUSED RECIPES

Here you will find a selection of great recipes that you can use to produce a variety of delicious edibles infused with CBD oil. We also provide a selection of tasty recipes for edible treats for your pets so that they too can enjoy the healing properties of CBD oil. And of course, you can make all these delicious recipes in the comfort of your own home.

CBD BUTTER

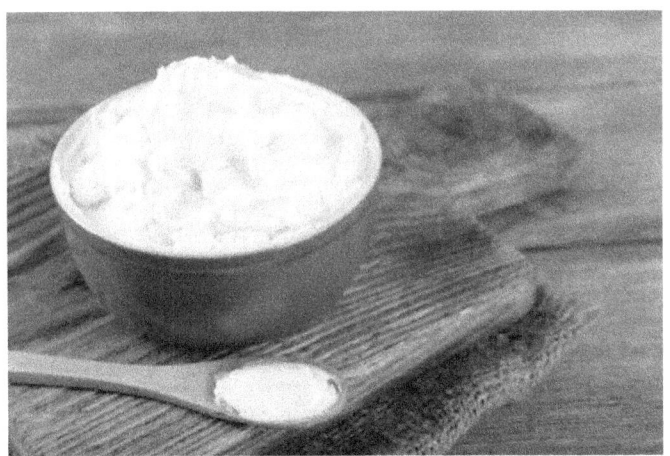

Ingredients:

- 2 cups salted or unsalted butter
- 1 cup filtered water
- 5/8-ounce CBD oil

Instructions:

1. Cut the butter into small cubes

2. Place the butter into a small pot with the water and add the oil

3. Heat for 2 hours over low heat, stirring frequently

4. Leave it to cool for a few minutes

5. Stir to combine the mixture and pour into a container, preferably airtight

6. Store in the refrigerator and use as you would normal butter.

GOLDEN MILK WITH CBD OIL

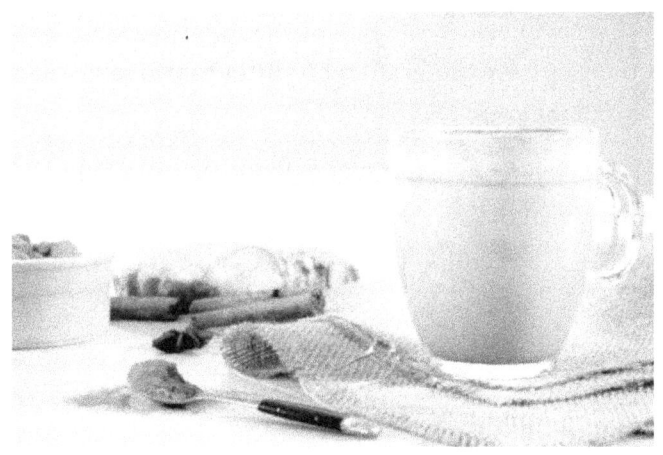

Ingredients:

- 2 cups of coconut or almond milk
- 1 tsp organic coconut oil
- 1 tsp curcumin (turmeric)

- ½ tsp cinnamon powder (Ceylon is best)
- 1 tsp raw honey or maple syrup
- ¼ tsp ginger powder or a 1-inch chunk of fresh ginger
- 1 tsp vanilla extract
- Pinch ground black pepper
- Pinch clove
- Pinch nutmeg
- .1-ounce CBD oil

Instructions:

1. Place the milk, spices and the vanilla into a small pan and heat gently for 10 minutes over a low heat

2. Remove the pan from the heat and transfer to two mugs; add the CBD oil and stir to combine

You can split the recipe in half if you only require one drink. You can also use Stevia in place of the syrup or honey.

CHOCOLATE LATTE WITH CBD OIL

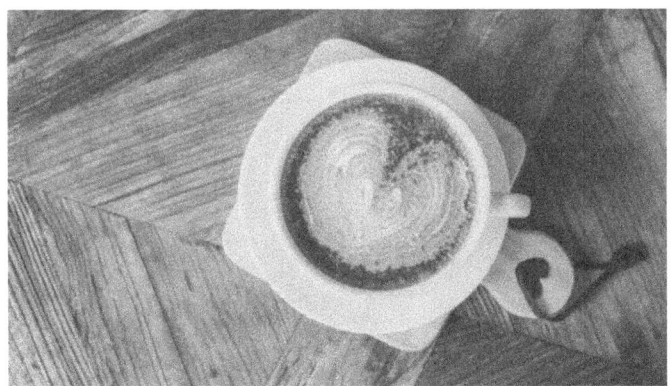

Ingredients:

- 1 cup unsweetened milk, plant-based – coconut, almond, etc.
- 1 tbsp raw cacao powder
- 1 tbsp organic maple syrup
- 1 tsp vanilla extract
- Pinch sea salt

- 1 dropper of neutral CBD oil – adjust according to taste
- Flavorings of your choice, i.e. a little cayenne and cinnamon, a dash of cardamom, a drop of rose water, fine ground culinary lavender, etc.

Instructions:

1. Mix all the ingredients together in a mall pot, leaving the CBD oil out

2. Over medium heat, bring the ingredients to a simmer, stirring to break lumps up

3. Remove from the heat and ad the CBD oil, whisking thoroughly

4. Serve hot or pour over ice

CHOCOLATE COCONUT FAT BOMBS WITH CBD OIL

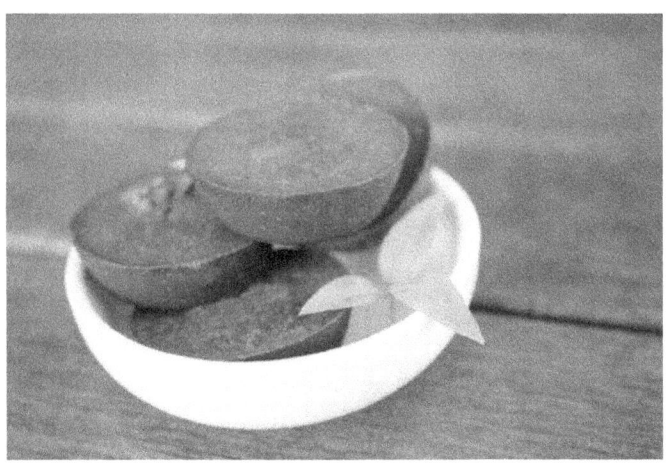

Ingredients:

- 1/3 to 2/3-ounce (to taste) CBD oil
- ½ cup coconut butter
- ½ cup coconut oil
- ½ cup raw cacao powder

- 1 tsp organic honey, or another organic sweetener (optional)

Instructions:

1. Melt the coconut oil over low heat until it has liquefied

2. Whisk in the cacao until all lumps are gone; if using sweetener, add now and stir until a smooth consistency is reached

3. Pour the mixture into 6 silicone muffin pan cups and refrigerate for about half an hour or until firm

4. Melt the coconut butter over low heat until it has just liquefied and then add the CBD oil, whisking thoroughly

5. Remove the chocolate mixture from the cups and spread the CBD and coconut mixture over the top of each one; refrigerate for another half hour or until firm enough.

Store in the refrigerator

PEPPERMINT CHOCOLATE CUPS WITH CBD OIL

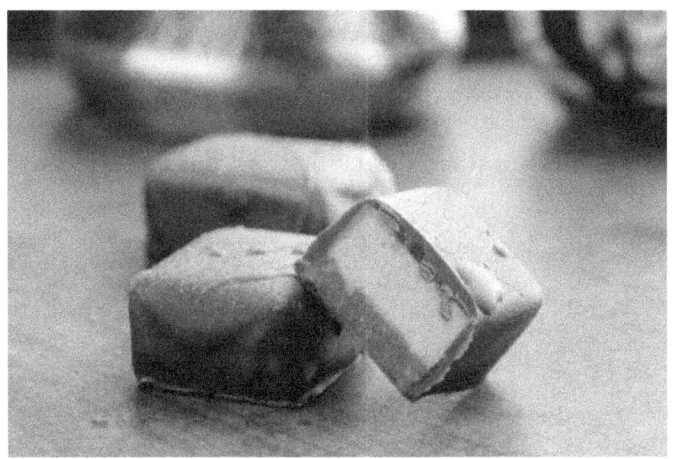

Ingredients:

- ¾ cup Rawmio mint chocolate*
- ¼ cup cacao butter
- 2 tbsp cashew butter

- ¼ cup coconut butter
- 1 tsp vanilla extract
- 2 tbsp organic maple syrup
- 1/8 tsp sea salt
- 1 ½ tsp CBD oil
- ¼ tsp spinach powder or green Matcha powder

* You can also use CBD dark chocolate or vegan chocolate chips (vegan) with a couple of drops of peppermint essence

Instructions:

1. Place the chocolate into the top half of a double boiler and melt to a smooth consistency

2. Divide the chocolate between 6 small molds (peanut butter cup molds) and freeze for about 10 minutes or until the chocolate is hard

3. Meanwhile, mix together the cashew, cacao, coconut butter, maple syrup, vanilla essence and sea salt in the top half of the double boiler and heat, whisking until you have a melted smooth consistency

4. Add the Matcha/spinach powder and the CBD oil whisking to blend thoroughly

5. Divide the mixture between the cups, pouring over the dark chocolate and freeze for about 20 minutes or until fully set

Store in the refrigerator

COOKIES, CREAM AND CBD OIL CHEESECAKE BITES

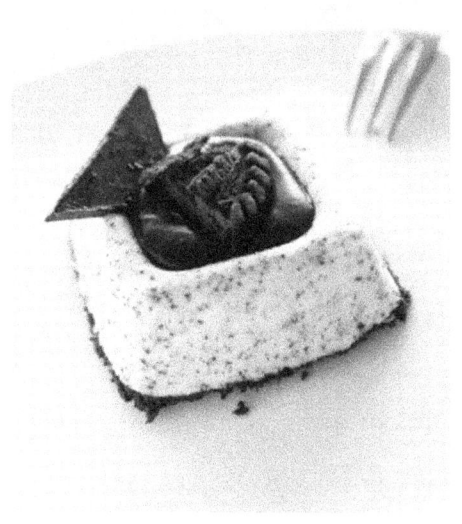

Ingredients:

For the Cookie Base:

- ½ cup fine almond flour
- 4 tbsp raw cacao powder
- ½ tsp 50% monk fruit extract
- 1 tsp baking powder, preferably gluten-free
- 1 flax egg – mix 1 tbsp flax seed with 3 tbsp water and mix thoroughly
- 1 tbsp ghee or coconut oil
- 5 drops stevia – vanilla cream

For the Cream Cheese Filling:

- ½ cup almond butter
- 1 cup plain cream cheese
- ¼ tsp 50% monk fruit extract
- Pinch vanilla bean powder
- 2 ½ to 5 droppers of CBD oil – start low and add if needed

Instructions:

To make the cookie base:

1. Preheat your oven to 300° F

2. Mix the almond flour, monk fruit, cacao powder, salt and baking powder together, whisking to thoroughly incorporate everything

3. Add the oil and the flax egg and stir to combine

4. Flatten the dough on a sheet of parchment paper and cut the cookies – they should be 1-2 inches across

5. Bake until crispy, around 12 to 15 minutes and leave them to cool to room temperature – as they cool, the cookies will crisp up. Once cooled and completely crispy, crumble them.

To make the cream cheese filling:

1. Put all the cream cheese filling ingredients together in a bowl and combine well – use an electric hand mixer to help you get the filling to a fluffy and smooth consistency

2. Fold half of the crumbled cookie mixture in

3. Now scoop the mixture, using an ice-cream scoop or cookie scoop and roll each one in the rest of the crumbled cookie mixture until coated

4. Refrigerate to firm them up

If you make a large batch, you can freeze them until you want them

CHOCOLATE CHIP COOKIES WITH CBD OIL

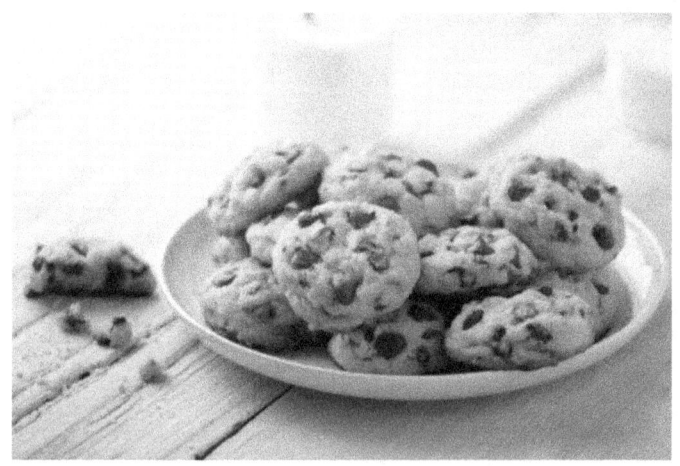

Ingredients:

- 3 tsp CBD oil (unflavored is best)
- 3 cups all-purpose flour
- 1 tsp baking soda
- 1 cup soft brown sugar

- 1 cup granulated white sugar
- ½ tsp salt
- 2 cups chocolate chips, semi-sweet are best
- 1 cup butter, softened
- 2 tsp vanilla extract
- 2 tsp hot water
- 2 eggs

Instructions:

1. Preheat the oven to 350° F

2. Mix together the brown and white sugars, the butter and the CBD oil until you have a creamy consistency

3. Beat the eggs into the mixture, add the vanilla extract and stir to combine

4. Add the flour gradually, stirring to combine

5. Put the baking soda in a small container and add the hot water, stirring until the soda has dissolved completely

6. Add the batter with the salt and stir until thoroughly distributed

7. Fold the chocolate chips into the mixture

8. Line a baking sheet with parchment paper and spoon out the batter, leaving a gap of 2 inches between each cookie

9. Bake for about 10 minutes or until the cookies are a golden-brown color

Leave to cool before serving

Store in an airtight container

GUACAMOLE DIP

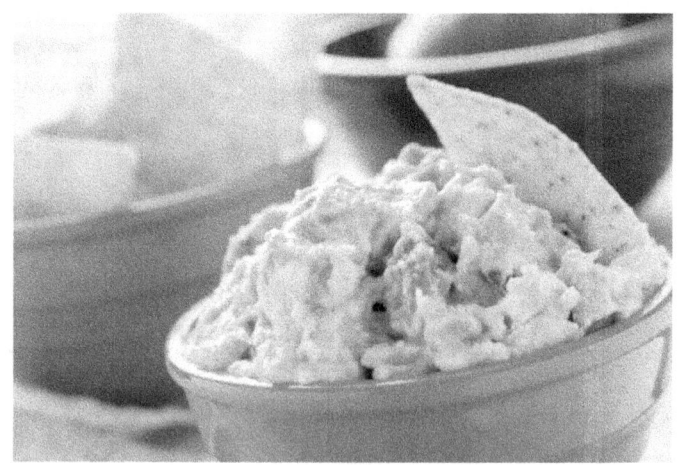

Ingredients:

- 3 whole avocados
- 1 tsp CBD oil
- 1 lime

- ½ cup onion, diced
- 1 tsp salt
- 2 Roma tomatoes, diced
- 3 tbs fresh cilantro, chopped
- 1 tsp garlic, minced

Instructions:

1. Slice the avocado in half, remove the stone and scoop the flesh into a bowl

2. Mash thoroughly

3. Extract the juice from the lime and add to the avocado with the salt and the CBD oil; stir to combine

4. Add the rest of the ingredients and stir

5. Season with salt, pepper, cayenne or whatever takes your fancy

6. Refrigerate until needed

STRAWBERRY AND CBD OIL VINAIGRETTE SALAD DRESSING

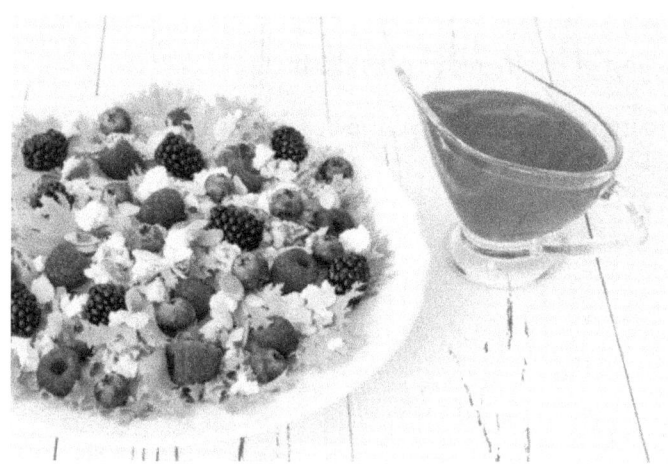

Ingredients:

- 1 cup fresh strawberries
- 1 tsp organic apple cider vinegar
- 2 tbsp red wine vinegar
- 3 tbsp extra virgin olive oil

- ½ dropper CBD oil

Instructions:

1. Place all of the ingredients into your blender

2. Blitz to a smooth consistency

3. Store in the refrigerator until needed

STRAWBERRY, ORANGE, AND CBD OIL SALAD DRESSING

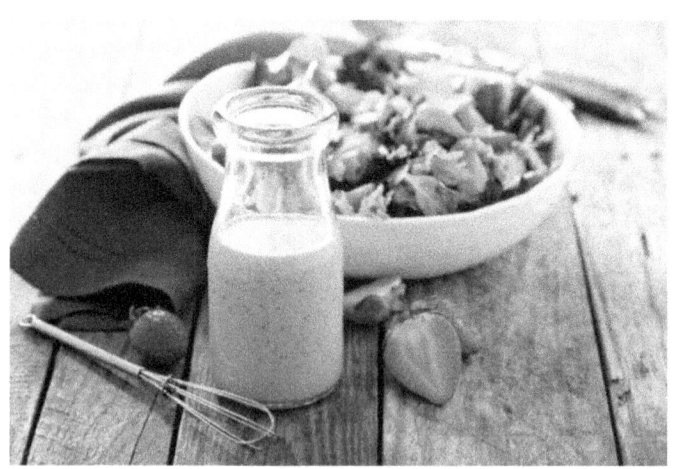

Ingredients:

- ¼ cup raspberry vinegar
- ½ cup pure orange juice
- ¼ cup extra virgin olive oil
- 2 tsp Dijon mustard

- 1 tbsp organic honey
- CBD oil to taste – start with a few drops and build up
- Salt and pepper for seasoning

Instructions:

1. Add all the ingredients to your blender

2. Blitz until you have a smooth consistency and taste; if more CBD is required, add and then blitz again

3. Store in the refrigerator

If you want more of a raspberry flavor, add a few raspberries to the blender before you blend.

COCONUT WATER ICE CUBES WITH CBD OIL

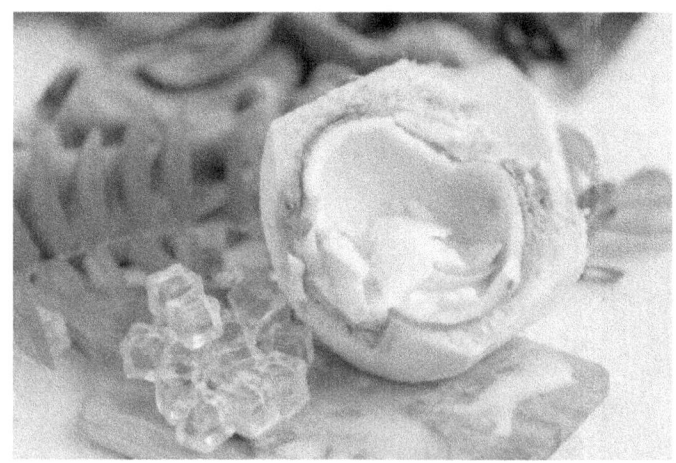

Ingredients:

- As much pure coconut water as it takes to fill your ice cube trays
- CBD oil

. . .

Instructions:

1. Pour the coconut water into a jug and add a few drops of CBD oil – do this to your taste, there is no set amount

2. Stir well to make sure the oil is distributed and pour into your ice cube trays

3. Freeze until needed

CBD GUMMIES

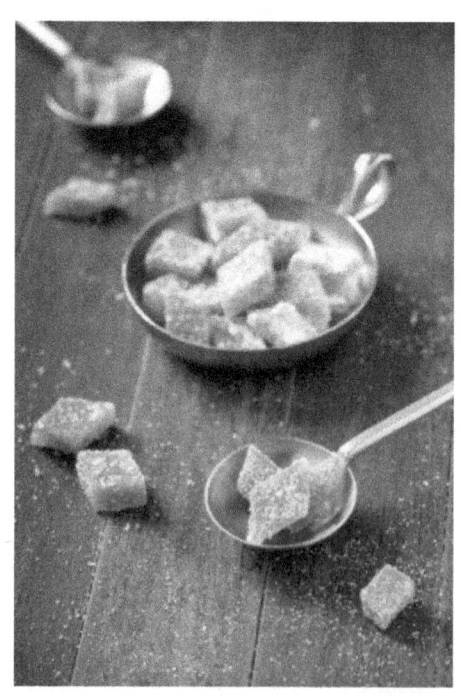

Ingredients:

- 1 cup tart cherry juice (or your preference)
- 2 tablespoons of gelatin
- 2 tablespoons of honey (or preferred sweetener)
- CBD oil

Instructions:

1. Pour the juice into a saucepan and bring it to a simmer over low heat.

2. Whisk in the gelatin and honey, stirring until everything is combined.

3. Turn off the heat and add your CBD oil. Stir once more to combine.

4. Pour the gelatin into whatever mold you're using. Place in the fridge or freezer to solidify.

5. If you like, you can roll the gummies in citric acid for a sour gummi.

CBD PARFAIT WITH HEMP MILK

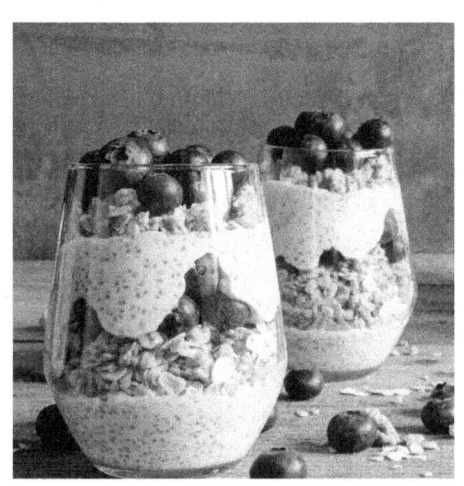

Ingredients:

- 2 cups of yogurt
- 1 cup of berries
- 1 cup of granola

- CBD oil to preference
- 2 tablespoons of chia seeds (optional)

Instructions:

1. Layer ½ cup of yogurt on the bottom of your glass.

2. Layer ¼ of granola over the yogurt.

3. ¼ of berries

4. 2-3 drops of CBD oil (or to your preference).

5. Repeat until the glass is full.

CBD PESTO PASTA WITH SHRIMP

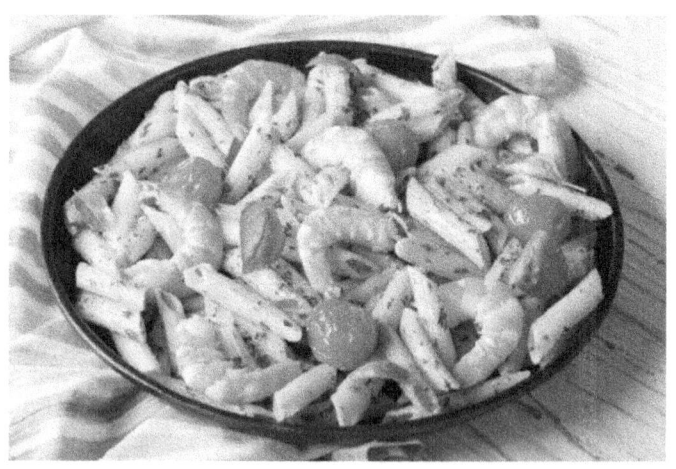

Ingredients for pesto:

- 2 cups of fresh baby spinach
- 1 cup of fresh basil
- ½ cup of fresh italian parsley
- ½ cup of cherry tomatoes

- 1 tablespoon of pine nuts
- 2 tablespoons of lemon juice
- 1/3 cup of grated Parmesan cheese
- 2 cloves of garlic
- 2 tablespoons of olive oil
- CBD oil to preference
- Salt and pepper to taste

Ingredients for pasta:

- 8 ounces of uncooked pasta
- 1 lb of fresh shrimp, peeled and deveined
- 1 lb of asparagus, cut into pieces
- ½ cup of cherry tomatoes, halved
- 2 tablespoons of butter
- 1 tablespoon of olive oil
- 1 tablespoon of lemon juice
- 1 teaspoon of red pepper flakes
- 1 teaspoon of cayenne (optional)
- Salt and pepper to taste

Instructions:

1. Place all of pesto ingredients in a blender. Blend until it is a smooth sauce.

2. Cook pasta according to package directions.

3. Place asparagus in the boiling pasta water for the last 3 or 4 minutes of

cooking. Drain and rinse with pasta.

4. Mix red pepper flakes, cayenne, salt, and pepper together.

5. Melt butter and heat oil in a skillet over medium heat. Dip each side of the shrimp in the seasoning mixture, then add to the skillet. Sprinkle with lemon juice and cook until pink on both sides.

6. Once the shrimp are cooked, add the asparagus and pasta to the skillet and saute for a moment. Remove from heat.

7. Add 6 to 8 tablespoons of pesto sauce to the pasta, depending on preference. Add the tomatoes and basil, then sprinkle with Parmesan.

CBD INFUSED PARMESAN MASHED POTATOES

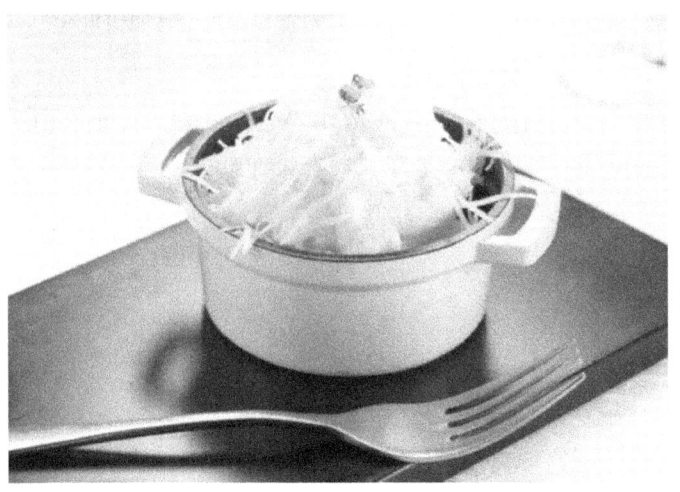

Ingredients:

- 4 lbs of potatoes
- A pinch of salt
- 2 cups of milk

- 5 tablespoons of butter
- 4 crushed garlic cloves
- CBD oil to preference
- grated Parmesan cheese

Instructions:

1. Peel and dice potatoes. Add water and a pinch of salt to a large pot, and bring to a boil. Add the potatoes to the boiling water, reduce heat to simmer and allow to boil for about 20 minutes.

2. While the potatoes are boiling, melt butter over low heat in a second saucepan. Add the CBD oil and stir. Then add milk, garlic, and pepper, then stir.

3. Reduce heat and allow to cook for 3 minutes before removing from heat.

4. When the potatoes are soft, drain the water and return to the pot. Add the butter and milk mixture, and mash the potatoes. Sprinkle with grated Parmesan.

CBD INFUSED STEAK AND VEGGIE BOWLS

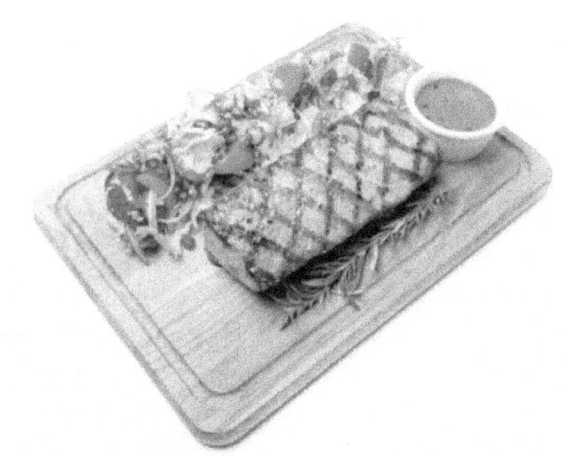

Ingredients:

- Steak, grilled and cut to your preference
- 2 tablespoons of olive oil
- ½ red onion, sliced thin
- 1 large sweet potato, cut into cubes

- 1 bundle of broccolini, stems removed and chopped
- 1 bundle of kale, stems removed
- 1 15 ounce can of chickpeas
- 1 teaspoon cumin
- 1 teaspoon chili powder
- garlic salt or garlic powder
- ¼ cup of tahini
- 1 tablespoon of agave
- juice of ½ lemon
- 2-4 tablespoons of hot water
- CBD oil to preference
- Salt and pepper to taste

Instructions:

1. Preheat your oven to 400°F.

2. Arrange the cubed sweet potatoes and sliced onions on a baking sheet, then drizzle oil over the top. Roast in oven for about 10 minutes. Take out, flip, and add more olive oil, then roast for another 10 minutes.

3. Heat a skillet over medium heat.

4. Add chickpeas and seasonings (cumin, chili powder, garlic salt, salt) and toss so the chickpeas are coated.

5. Once the skillet has reached heat, add a tablespoon of oil and the chickpeas. Let them saute, stirring constantly. They should brown gradually for about 10 minutes. Remove from heat.

6. Once the sweet potatoes and broccolini have roasted for about 20

minutes, add the kale and drizzle more oil over the leaves. Season with salt and pepper, and roast for another 4 minutes.

7. In a mixing bowl, combine tahini, lemon juice, and agave, then mix to combine. Add hot water a tablespoon at a time, until it thins to a pourable sauce.

8. Divide vegetables between bowls, then layer chickpeas and steak on top. Add a generous amount of sauce.

CBD INFUSED MOZZARELLA STUFFED MEATBALLS

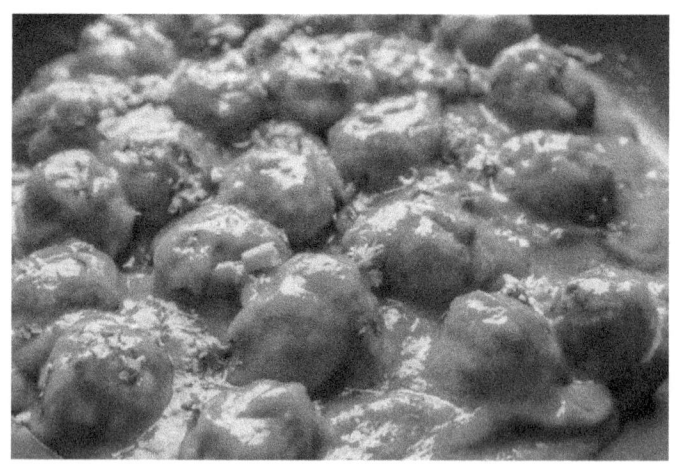

Ingredients:

- 7 cups of crushed tomatoes
- ½ cup of onion
- 2 cloves of garlic, chopped
- 2 teaspoons of dried basil

- 1 teaspoon of pepper
- 1 teaspoon of salt
- 1 lb of beef
- 1 lb of mild sausage
- 1 cup of breadcrumbs
- 1 teaspoon of onion powder
- 1 teaspoon of garlic powder
- 1 teaspoon of thyme
- 1 teaspoon of oregano
- 2 eggs
- 4 mozzarella sticks (string cheese), cut into 5 even pieces
- CBD oil to preference

Instructions:

1. Add the crushed tomatoes, ½ cup of onion, chopped garlic, basil, and ½ teaspoon each of salt and pepper in a slow cooker. Set the cooker on high and allow to cook for about a half hour while making the meatballs.

2. In a large mixing bowl, combine beef, sausage, breadcrumbs, onion powder, garlic powder, thyme, oregano, eggs, CBD oil, and ½ teaspoon each of salt and pepper. Use your hands to mix everything together so the ingredient are evenly distributed.

3. Form a ball about 1 ½ inch diameter ball from the meatball mixture. Press a piece of mozzarella into the middle, surrounding it with the meatball mixture. Continue until all the meat mixture is used.

4. Add the meatballs to the slow cooker. Cook for 2 to 2 ½ hours on high, until the meatballs are cooked through.

CBD INFUSED CHICKEN PENNE ALFREDO

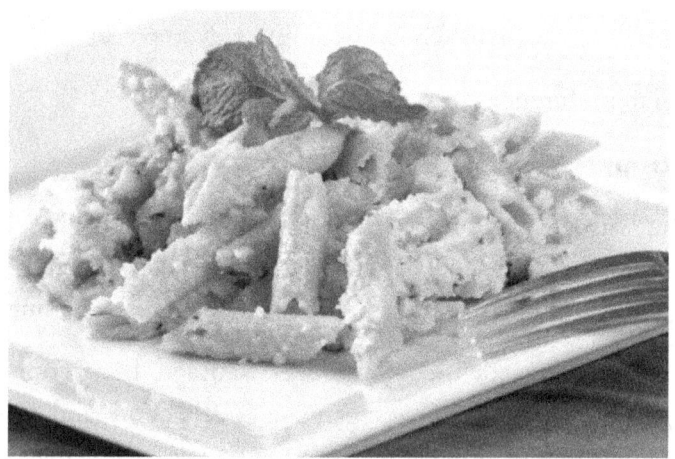

Ingredients:

- 4 tablespoons of butter
- 1 ½ lbs of chicken, cut into pieces
- 1 teaspoon of salt

- 1 teaspoon of pepper
- 1 teaspoon of oregano
- 1 teaspoon of basil
- ¼ cup of parsley
- 4 cloves of minced garlic
- 3 tablespoons of flour
- 2 cups of milk
- 1 cup of parmesan cheese, grated
- 16 ounces of penne pasta

Instructions:

1. Heat 1/2 tablespoon of butter in a large skillet over medium-low heat. Once melted, add the chicken, add ½ teaspoon of salt, pepper, oregano, and basil. Cook until the chicken is cooked through (no longer pink, with clear juices). Remove from skillet and set aside.

2. Heat 2 tablespoons over medium-low heat in the same skillet. Add minced garlic and 1 ½ tablespoons of flour. Cook until the garlic is soft and fragrant.

3. Add the remainder of the flour, and then slowly add the milk, stirring as you do.

4. Add the remaining ½ teaspoon of salt, pepper, oregano, and basil. Add ½ cup of parmesan to the skillet, also. Add the amount of CBD oil you prefer. Stir to combine.

Cook pasta according to package directions and drain. Combine the cheese sauce with the chicken and pasta, stirring. Top with the remaining ½ cup of parmesan.

CBD CHAMOMILE TEA LATTE

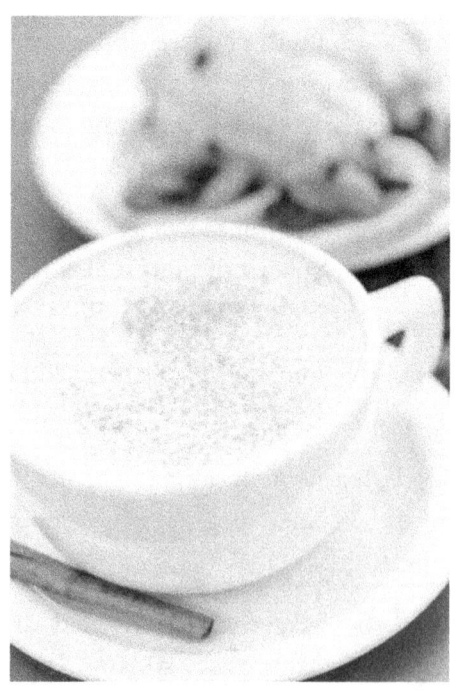

Ingredients:

- 2 cups of unsweetened almond milk
- 2 chamomile tea bags or 2 tablespoons of loose leaf tea
- 2 tablespoons of maple syrup
- CBD oil to preference
- ⅛ teaspoon of ground ginger
- ⅛ teaspoon of ground nutmeg

Instructions:

1. Heat the milk and tea in a saucepan, but do not let it boil.

2. Remove the tea and whisk in the CBD oil, nutmeg, ginger, and maple syrup.

Add froth to to your taste.

CBD GOLDEN MILK POPSICLES

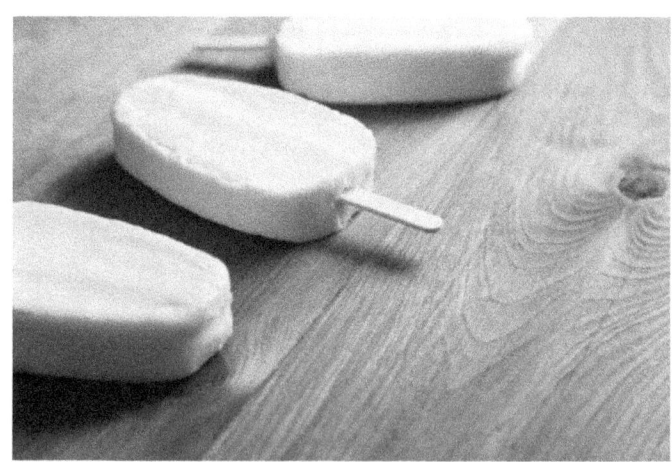

Ingredients:

- 1 14 ounce can of full fat coconut milk, shaken to mix solid and liquid
- ⅓ cup of nut milk
- ½ teaspoon of vanilla
- ⅓ cup of honey

- ¼ teaspoon of ginger
- CBD oil to preference
- 1 tablespoon of coconut milk powder

Instructions:

1. Pour all of the ingredients into a saucepan. Heat over medium-low heat, stirring until the mixture is smooth and ingredients combined.

2. Pour the mixture into popsicle molds and allow to freeze for at least 3 hours before eating.

CBD ICED COFFEE

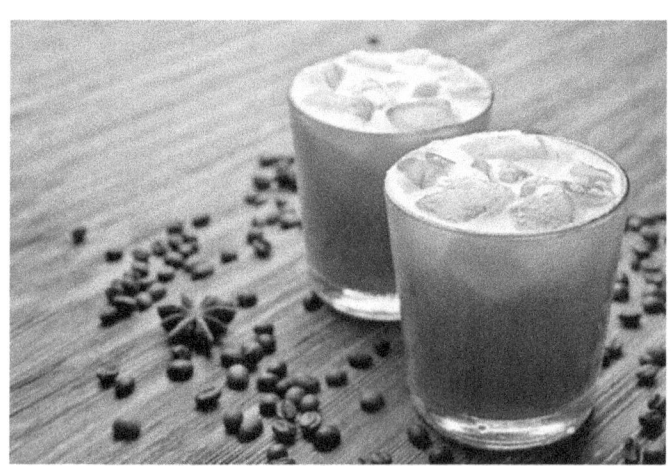

Ingredients:

- One pitcher of coffee prepared as you prefer, with whatever additions you like (milk, cream, sugar, etc.), allowed to cool

- CBD oil to your preference

Instructions:

1. Add the CBD oil to the cold coffee and stir to distribute evenly.

2. Pour part of the coffee into ice cube trays and freeze.

3. Place frozen coffee cubes in glass and pour coffee over the top.

CBD MARGARITA

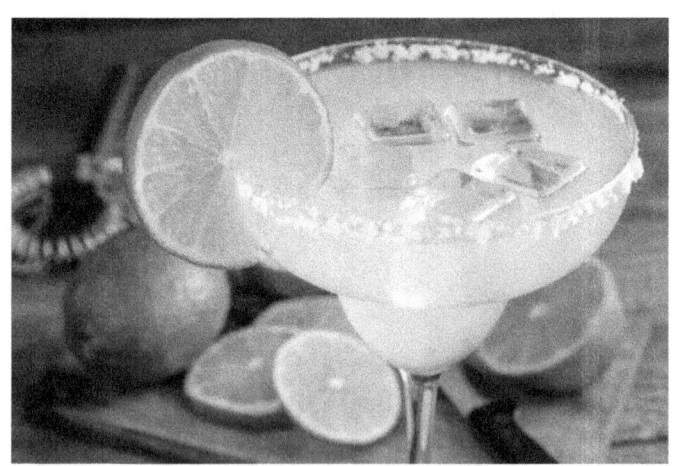

Ingredients:

- 1 ounce of mezcal
- 1 ounce of aquavit
- ¾ ounce of lime juice
- ¾ ounce of agave syrup

- 1 ounce of green juice (celery, arugula, kale, etc.)
- 1 pinch of sea salt
- CBD oil to preference

Instructions:

1. In a shaker filled with ice, combine the mezcal, aquavit, lime juice, agave syrup, green juice, salt, and CBD oil.

2. Shake, then strain into a glass with ice cubes.

CHICKEN SALAD WITH CBD LEMON DRESSING

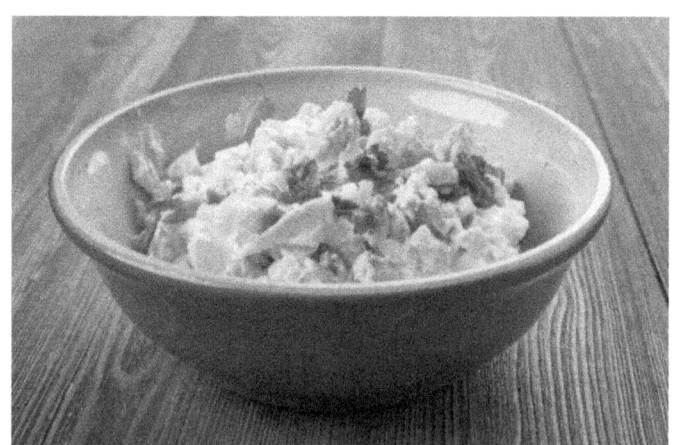

Ingredients:

- 2 tablespoons of olive oil
- 4 chicken thighs, skinless, boneless, and slice into pieces
- 1 tablespoon of Dijon mustard
- zest and juice of 1 lemon

- CBD oil to preference
- ¼ cup of mayonnaise
- 2 cloves of garlic, chopped
- 1 sliced avocado
- ½ of a cucumber, sliced
- ½ cup of sliced radishes

Instructions:

1. Rub the chicken thighs with the olive oil.

2. Heat a frying pan to medium-high heat. Fry the chicken in the pan, turning regularly to cook evenly. Once cooked through, set aside to cool.

3. In a mixing bowl, mix the Dijon mustard, lemon juice and zest. Then add the mayo and garlic, then the CBD oil. Stir until completely combined and emulsified.

Add the cucumber, radishes, and avocado along with whatever other vegetables you enjoy. Mix to combine, then fold in the chicken pieces.

CBD CHILI CON CARNE

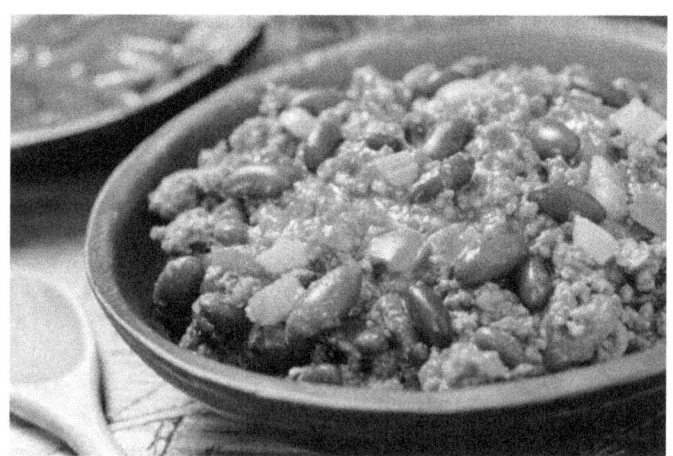

Ingredients:

- 2 15 ounce cans of black beans, drained
- 1 can of black eyed peas, drained
- 2 15 ounce cans of red kidney beans, drained
- 2 medium sweet onions, chopped

- 8-12 plum tomatoes, chopped
- ⅓ cup of red wine
- 1 ½ lbs of ground beef
- 2 cloves of garlic, minced
- 2 tablespoons of cumin
- 2 tablespoons of chili powder
- 1 tablespoon of chili flakes
- 3 tablespoons of Worcestershire sauce
- CBD oil to preference

Instructions:

1. Put all the beans in a large pot over low heat. When they are heated through and steam begins to rise, add the red wine, cumin, chili powder, chili flakes, and Worcestershire sauce. Stir to combine.

2. Let it cook for about 30 minutes, then add the onions and tomatoes.

3. Heat a frying pan or skillet to medium heat. Add the ground beef and garlic, then cook until brown, stirring regularly. Add the browned beef to the beans and vegetables.

4. Add the CBD oil. Let it cook for 1 to 2 hours, then serve.

CBD BROWNIES

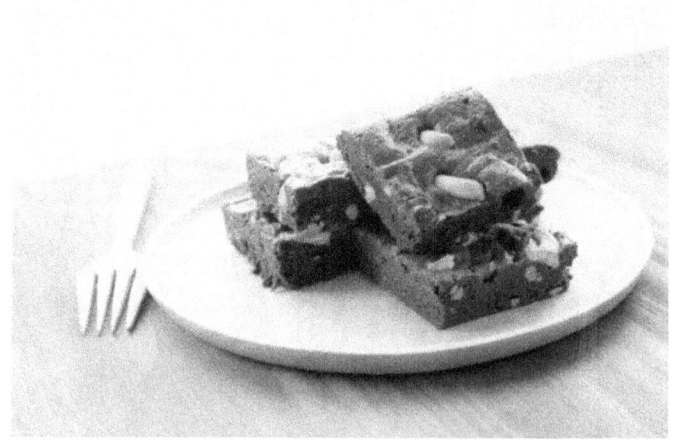

Ingredients:

- ½ cup of CBD butter (recipe above)
- 1 cup of sugar
- 1 tablespoon of vanilla extract
- 2 eggs

- ½ cup of all-purpose flour
- ½ cup of cacao powder
- ¼ teaspoon of baking powder
- ¼ teaspoon of salt
- Nuts

Instructions:

1. Preheat your oven to 350 °F. Prepare a square baking pan with parchment paper and/or cooking spray.

2. In a saucepan over medium-low heat, melt butter. Stir in sugar until combined.

3. Pour the butter mixture into a mixing bowl, then add and combine the eggs and vanilla.

4. Mix in the baking powder, cacao, flour, and salt.

5. Spread the batter into the prepared pan and top with whatever nuts you prefer.

Bake for 25 or 30 minutes, until a toothpick stuck into the middle comes out clean.

CBD FRESH MINT TEA

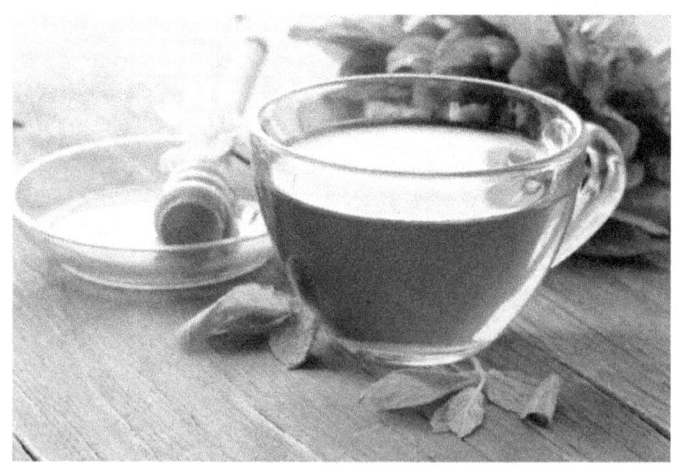

Ingredients:

- 2 handfuls of fresh mint leaves
- 4 cups of water
- Squeeze of lemon
- 2 cups of honey

- CBD oil to preference

Instructions:

1. Using a double boiler, heat the honey. Alternatively, boil water in a large saucepan and then place a small saucepan in the boiling water. Place the honey in the smaller saucepan.

2. Add the CBD oil to the honey and stir until fully combined. Remove from heat and allow to cool.

3. Heat the water to about 190°F. Alternatively, heat to boiling and then allow to cool for 2 to 3 minutes.

4. Place the mint leaves in a glass container. Pour the hot water over the top of the leaves. Allow to steep.

5. Add honey and lemon to taste.

CH. 7: PET EDIBLES AND TREATS

Your pets deserve to experience the benefits of CBD oil too and while there are plenty of places online that you can purchase CBD pet treats from, you could also consider making your own. Not only is this option cheaper, but you can also change the recipes to suit your pets. Be aware that while you can use human CBD oil, it is best to use pet-friendly oil as it has been specially formulated for animals.

As stated in a previous chapter on this subject, when you do decide to introduce CBD oil to your pet's diet, you should always use a carrier oil, such as coconut oil or bake them into treats, to make it more palatable for your pet.

As well, I will reiterate that it is prudent to start with a small dose of CBD oil based on your pet's size, administered in dropper form, sublingually, or by baking it into treats. You can consult with a CBD hemp oil specialist or a veterinarian that is open to holistic treatments. They can monitor your pet for changes, as well as provide guidance on how much CBD oil you should give your pet.

PEANUT BUTTER AND HONEY TREAT WITH CBD OIL

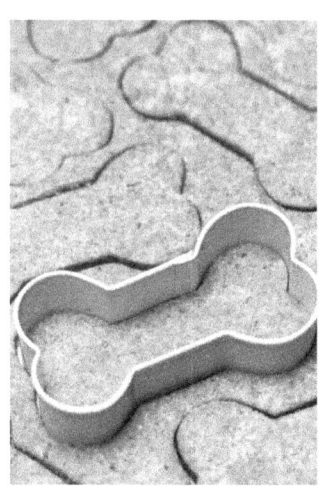

Ingredients:

- ⅔ cup of coconut oil
- ½ cup of peanut butter
- ¼ cup of honey

- 1 cup of rolled oats
- 1 cup of chicken broth
- 1 cup of whole wheat flour
- 1 cup of all-purpose flour
- 1 teaspoon of CBD oil

Instructions:

1. Preheat your oven to 350°F.

2. In a large mixing bowl, whisk together the coconut oil, peanut butter, honey, chicken broth, and CBD oil.

3. In a separate bowl, mix the two flours and add the oats.

4. Add the dry ingredients to the wet ingredients and fold them together.

5. Prepare a floured surface. Roll the dough out to a thickness of about ¼ of an inch.

6. Cut out treats using a cookie cutter.

7. Place on a baking sheet and bake for about 15 minutes. Let them cool before giving them to your furry friend.

GRAIN-FREE PEANUT BUTTER AND APPLESAUCE CBD OIL TREATS

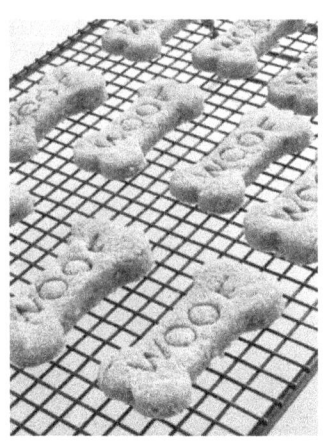

Ingredients:

- 1 tsp pet-friendly CBD oil
- ½ cup smooth peanut butter
- 1 ½ cups coconut flour
- 4 eggs

- ½ cup coconut oil

- 1 cup unsweetened applesauce

Instructions:

1. Preheat your oven to 350° F

2. Place all the ingredients together in a bowl and mix together; use an electric hand-mixer with dough hooks to make it easier

3. Form the dough into one large ball using your hands and place it between two sheets of baking paper

4. Roll it out to around ¼ inch thick

5. Using a small cookie cutter, cut out the treats and place them onto a lined baking tray

6. Bake for around 12 to 15 minutes and then turn out onto a cooling rack

FROZEN YOGURT AND PEANUT BUTTER TREATS

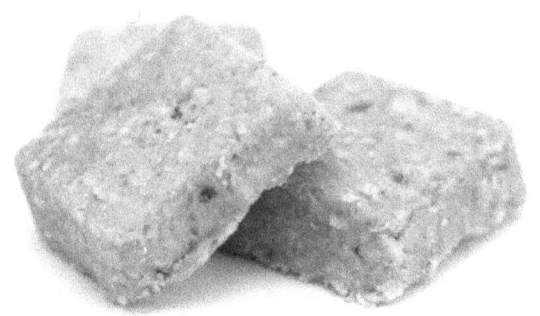

Ingredients:

- 1 cup of peanut butter
- 32 ounces of vanilla yogurt
- CBD oil

Instructions:

1. Microwave peanut butter on high for about 30 seconds, then stir. Continue until the peanut butter has melted and can be easily poured.

2. Add the yogurt and CBD oil. Stir thoroughly so the CBD is evenly distributed.

3. Pour the mixture into molds or an ice cube tray. Freeze for about 2 hours or until they are solid.

NO BAKE COCONUT AND CBD TREATS

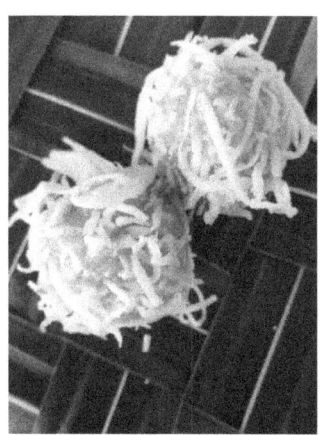

Ingredients:

- 2 ½ cups of rolled oats
- ⅓ cup of coconut oil
- 3 tablespoons of peanut butter
- 1 teaspoon of CBD oil

- ½ cup of shredded coconut

Instructions:

1. Mix the rolled oats, peanut butter, CBD oil, and coconut oil together. A food processor will make it easier.

2. Roll the mixture into small balls. The larger the ball, the larger the dose of CBD.

3. Roll the balls in the shredded coconut until it's covered completely.

Place on a baking sheet lined with parchment paper and chill for 30 minutes, until solidified.

SWEET POTATO AND CBD TREATS

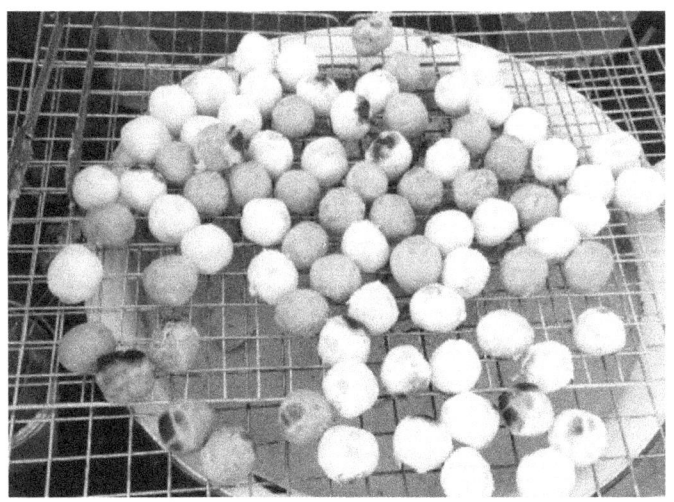

Ingredients:

- 2 medium sweet potatoes, peeled, baked, and mashed
- ½ cup of coconut flour
- ½ cup of coconut oil or bacon grease

- 1 egg
- 1 teaspoon of CBD oil
- 1 to tablespoons of water

Instructions:

1. Preheat your oven to 350°F.

2. Mix all the ingredients together thoroughly. You made need to add extra flour to reach a thick consistency.

3. Form into balls about 1 inch in diameter.

4. Place on baking sheet lined with parchment paper.

5. Let bake for 20 minutes or so. Let them cool completely before giving them to your pup.

FROZEN PUMPKIN AND CBD TREATS

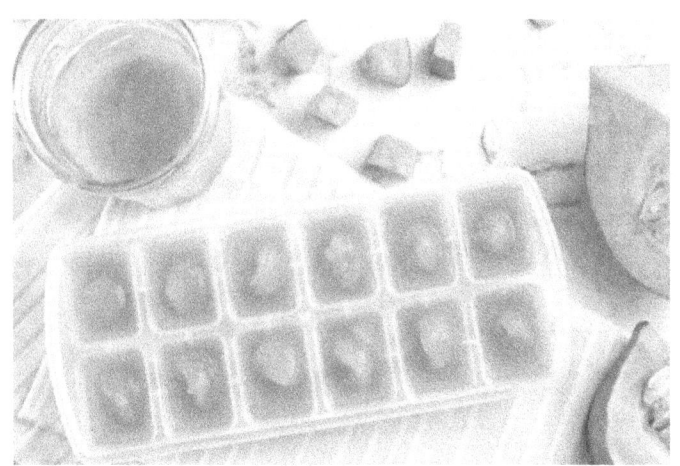

Ingredients:

- 1 cup of pumpkin puree
- ½ cup of unflavored yogurt
- 1 teaspoon of CBD oil

Instructions

1. Mix the ingredients together thoroughly.

2. Pour the mixture into an ice cube tray.

3. Freeze for at least 2 hours.

4. Keep in freezer so they don't melt.

Start off with small amounts of the CBD oil, especially if your dog or cat has never had a CBD Oil-infused edible before, and then gradually increase the amount in each recipe.

CONCLUSION

By now, you should have a total understanding of the ECS and how cannabinoids like those found in CBD hemp oil interact with the body. Whether you consider yourself in good health or you are struggling with anxiety, chronic pain, or another condition, CBD oil offers benefits that promote total wellness. Your body will have a better chance of fighting off stress and illness while encouraging the body to remain in a state of balance.

Keep in mind that the results you experience from CBD hemp oil depend on the number of receptors in your body, as well as the potency of the extract, your individual dosage, and how long you have been taking it. It takes time for the number of receptors to increase, so do not expect the full results immediately after starting your regimen.

By sourcing CBD hemp oil from a reputable company, as well as by choosing an organic brand with third-party testing you can ensure you are putting nothing but the beneficial ingredients in your body. I believe that this book provides you with all the information you need to try CBD oil for the first time and experience its full range of benefits.

Best of luck!

. . .

Finally, if you enjoyed this book, then I would like to ask you for a favor. Would you be kind enough to leave a review for this book on Amazon? It would be greatly appreciated.

Click here to leave a review for this book on Amazon

Take care and best regards,

Terry Gordon

REFERENCES

https://www.forbes.com/sites/monazhang/2018/04/05/no-cbd-is-not-legal-in-all-50-states/#1ba46d4c762c

https://hempmedspx.com/states-cbd-oil-legal-purchase/

https://www.medicalmarijuanainc.com/what-is-cbd-oil/

https://www.solcbd.com/blogs/news/using-cbd-oil-for-epilepsy

http://adai.uw.edu/marijuana/factsheets/cannabinoids.htm

http://norml.org/library/item/introduction-to-the-endocannabinoid-system

https://www.organicfacts.net/health-benefits/oils/cbd-oil-benefits-uses-side-effects.html

http://www.advancedholistichealth.org/history.html

https://hightimes.com/sponsored/cbd-hemp-oil-benefits-is-it-legal-and-recent-news/

https://healthyhempoil.com/cannabidiol-legal-status/

https://greenrushdaily.com/what-is-the-endocannabinoid-system/

http://canorml.org/cbd.html

https://www.medicalmarijuanainc.com/what-is-cbd-hemp-oil/

https://healthyhempoil.com/hemp-cbd-vs-cannabis-cbd/

https://hempmedspx.com/about-Hemp-Stalk-Oil/

http://www.ncsl.org/research/agriculture-and-rural-development/state-industrial-hemp-statutes.aspx

https://www.ncbi.nlm.nih.gov/pmc/articles/PMC2241751/

http://normltn.org/does-breast-milk-contain-cannabinoids/

https://sensiseeds.com/en/blog/cannabinoid-science-101-what-is-anandamide/

https://cbdoilreview.org/cbd-cannabidiol/cbd-benefits/

https://www.ncbi.nlm.nih.gov/pubmed/22716160

https://www.medicalmarijuanainc.com/where-can-i-buy-cbd-hemp-oil/

https://healthyhempoil.com/buy-cannabidiol-guide/

https://www.verywellmind.com/what-does-a-marijuana-high-feel-like-22303

https://www.organicfacts.net/health-benefits/oils/cbd-oil-benefits-uses-side-effects.html#cite-link-17

https://elixinol.com/education/faqs/

https://www.projectcbd.org/guidance/conditions

https://highlandpharms.com/faq-cbd-hemp-oil/#1520973857483-3052f361-95fa

https://elixinolcbd.com/blogs/buyers-guide/15974795-how-to-buy-cbd-oil-watch-out-for-these-3-traps

https://hightimes.com/sponsored/cbd-oil-legal-high-quality/

https://www.medicalmarijuanainc.com/cbd-hemp-oil-frequently-asked-questions/

https://www.marijuanatimes.org/the-endocannabinoid-system-a-history-of-endocannabinoids-and-cannabis/

https://kidshealth.org/en/parents/breast-bottle-feeding.html

https://www.cancer.gov/about-cancer/understanding/statistics

https://www.leafscience.com/2014/10/15/highest-cbd-strains/

https://www.marijuanabreak.com/best-cbd-oils-pain-relief

http://www.hempoilfacts.com/wp-content/uploads/2016/05/SUCCESSFUL-THERAPY-OF-TREATMENT-RESISTANT-ADULT-ADHD-WITH-CANNABIS.pdf

http://www.hempoilfacts.com/cannabidiol-cbd-add-adhd-research/

https://www.medicaljane.com/2012/12/20/cannabidiol-cbd-medicine-of-the-future/

http://www.hempoilfacts.com/cannabidiol-cbd-arthritis-research/

https://www.healthline.com/health/migraine/cbd-oil-for-migraines#how-it-works

https://naturalwellnesscbdoil.com/cbd-oil-for-glaucoma-does-it-really-work/

https://www.whatiscbd.com/cbd-for-parkinsons-disease/

https://cbdinstead.com/blogs/cbd-senior-care/cbd-and-bone-health

https://ministryofhemp.com/blog/cbd-and-depression/

https://www.leafly.com/news/health/cbd-for-treating-anxiety

https://www.leafly.com/news/health/cbd-weight-loss-metabolism

https://www.ncbi.nlm.nih.gov/pubmed/22520455

https://www.ncbi.nlm.nih.gov/pubmed/850145

https://allcbdoilbenefits.com/epilepsy/

https://www.ncbi.nlm.nih.gov/pubmed/7413719

https://ministryofhemp.com/blog/cbd-for-schizophrenia/

https://www.ncbi.nlm.nih.gov/pubmed/24353209

https://cbdinstead.com/blogs/cbd-and-cardiovascular/3-big-ways-cbd-helps-with-heart-disease

https://www.medicaljane.com/2013/07/19/cbd-gives-birth-to-new-neurons-in-the-brain-2/

https://cheefbotanicals.com/using-cbd-oil-for-diabetes/

https://www.royalqueenseeds.com/blog-how-cbd-can-spice-up-your-sex-life-n1012

https://www.leafly.com/news/health/how-cannabis-helps-relieve-menopause-symptoms

https://www.compassionatecertificationcenters.com/the-potential-benefits-of-cbd-for-the-symptoms-of-bipolar-disorder/

https://cannabismd.com/health/mental/cbd-oil-for-the-treatment-of-bipolar-disorder/

http://www.marijuanatimes.org/how-cbds-can-effectively-treat-bipolar-disorder-symptoms-and-manic-episodes/

https://ministryofhemp.com/blog/cbd-cooking/

https://blog.bulletproof.com/cbd-oil-recipes-1b2b4c4t/

https://healthyhempoil.com/how-to-make-your-own-cbd-edibles/

https://healthyhempoil.com/cbd-for-pets-what-you-need-to-know/

https://healthyhempoil.com/5-cbd-treat-recipes-your-dog-will-love/

https://phytoanimalhealth.com/cbd-infused-dog-treats/

https://www.cleaneatingkitchen.com/cbd-gummies-sleep-hemp/

https://purehempbotanicals.com/cooking-with-cbd-pre-workout-vegan-parfait/

https://www.theherbsomm.com/single-post/Cooking-for-Wellness-Two-CBD-Recipes

https://www.endoca.com/blog/christmas-recipes-special-cbd-mashed-potatoes

https://www.thecbdistillery.com/cooking-with-cbd/

https://www.thecbdistillery.com/cooking-with-cbd/

https://www.thecbdistillery.com/cooking-with-cbd/

https://helloglow.co/cbd-recipes/slide/3

https://www.diamondcbd.com/blog/top-5-cbd-dishes-exciting-cbd-recipes-sweet-savory

https://goop.com/recipes/up-in-smoke/

https://premiumjane.com/blog/best-cbd-based-recipes/

http://420foodieclub.com/recipe/cbd-brownies/

http://420foodieclub.com/recipe/cbd-fresh-mint-tea/

https://premiumjane.com/blog/best-cbd-based-recipes

www.ingramcontent.com/pod-product-compliance
Lightning Source LLC
Chambersburg PA
CBHW070437180526
45158CB00019B/1473